Live, Work, Love

Live, Work, Love

LIVE
Work
LOVE

#Add**10**QualityYears

TERRY WILLIAMS

Live, Work, Love

A brain-based boss book

Published in 2017 by brainbasedboss.com

Auckland, New Zealand

ISBN: 978-1523208098

Live, Work, Love

Contents:

1

Why Am I Here and
Why Should I Care?

Our longevity, health and quality of life are due 30% to genetic luck and 70% to our choices and behaviours. We're dealt some cards and this book is about how to play the best hand, given those cards we've been dealt. No one wants to live forever but most of us would like to get the most out of whatever we've got coming. The vast majority of us would like to keep on going until we don't, not taper off to a long unhealthy tail of life. Regardless of how long we have, how do we stay healthier longer, optimise our happiness and make it all worthwhile?

There's a 2-panel cartoon I share often. The first panel is headed 1990 and features a skinny guy with a fat TV. The second panel is headed 2011 and features a fat guy with a skinny TV. That, in a nutshell, is symbolic of many of today's problems of affluence. This book suggests a toolbox of solutions.

If ever you're presenting information to anyone, your audience needs you to answer two questions quickly. Whether it's a sales pitch, staff meeting, job interview, blind date or this book, those questions are:

- Why am I here?

- Why should I care?

You are here reading because you are working, have or plan a family, and have goals like paying off a mortgage, fulfilling some dreams and being happy. You should care because, despite living in a country, and at a time, with unprecedented abundance and the longest life expectancies in human history, you would like to optimise your chances of living longer and better, not for the sake of merely sticking around but for that dreams / goals / happiness / family thing. Cancers, Diabetes, Heart disease and Lung disease will be what kills 9/10 people in industrialised nations and many of those are entirely preventable. Your health, longevity and productivity are due to 30% genetic luck and 70% your own lifestyle choices – choices you make (and don't make) many times every day. You also model those choices to your kids.

Work for you is not merely a pay packet. Your work, your *career*, says something about you and it is one way you make your mark in this world. Living longer and better would give you more chances to produce a legacy for your family and yourself. The example you set and the resources you provide will set your family up with a great platform to do even better.

OK, that's why you're here and why you should care. Why am I here with you and why do I care?

In addition to being a business speaker, trainer and author, I also dabble as a professional stand-up comedian. My most recent one-man stand-up comedy show 'The Grin Reaper' was in the 2013 New Zealand International Comedy Festival.

The show is primarily an hour of jokes and stories and it was themed around living longer. I drew on a few of the resources I cite in this book and wrote jokes and stories around those. At the end of the show, my conclusion was that the best thing you could do to add ten quality years to your life, and the lives of those you love, was to have a drink and prepare a meal with friends and family every day after a hard but productive workday, then enjoy that meal with those same people having a laugh, reflecting on the day and the past, and talking about plans for the future. I thanked my sponsors, gave away the prize bottles of Oyster Bay Sparkling Cuvee Brut, pointed them at www.thegrinreaper.co.nz and yelled, "Thank you. Goodnight!"

The show sold out, didn't lose me money, got great feedback online and in person from those attending, and received glowing reviews. Those were my goals for the production, yet they were all still very pleasant surprises. But the real surprise for me was the approaches from people afterwards. After a cursory complimentary comment, many people were genuinely and actively intrigued and interested in the concepts I'd been talking about – the serious concepts behind the humour. What books had I read? What was that website with the online life expectancy quiz I mentioned? How am I so thin and energetic at my age?

Subsequently and unrelated, I delivered a series of non-comedy business presentations about building winning teams around New Zealand in 2013 to over 6000 business leaders in 25 cities. In passing, I mentioned about my comedy show and its subject matter. Of the subsequent bookings I got following that series of presentations from audience members, two thirds of them were to perform my comedy show in conjunction with some local fundraising efforts. They wanted to know, and felt their people needed to know, about how to live better and longer. They especially liked the inter-relatedness of life and work and, much to my astonishment... love.

Clearly, there was a lot of curiosity around the overlap of these three aspects. These weren't hippies; these were bosses of organisations big and small, public and private, entrepreneurial and not-for-profit. My second book 'The Brain-Based Boss' about employee motivation and engagement had just been published and if enough book-buying business people start telling you that you should write a book about the subject of adding quality years to your life and working life, the message quickly gets through.

The timing is good. New Zealand and much of the rest of the world are wrestling with predictions of unsustainable pensions and superannuation budgets as the demographic bulge of baby boomers hits the arbitrary age of entitlement. People are living much longer than we used to when these lines in the sands of time of 60 or 65 were drawn. Should that age of entitlement be raised? Should payments be lowered? What about the burden to society of the billowing medical costs of the increasingly greying population? Could some tweaking make it work if people could opt for different starting ages of entitlement with lower amounts of payment the earlier they started? Will our voluntary compulsion to keep working and remain productive offset the economic demands of a greying population?

Uncertainty reigns and that's never good for individuals, countries or money.

Is it about the quantity of life or the quality of life? Well, if you're dead, the quality sucks.

I hate the term work-life balance. To me, it implies that there is this separate thing called 'work' and another separate thing called 'life' and they're in conflict with each other and mutually exclusive and to over-engage in one will be at the cost of the other, generating unhealthy anxiety and stress. I reject that linear and binary model in favour of a venn diagram of three intersecting spheres: life, work and love.

There's an overlap that shifts as we search for it and as we progress through life's stages. If technology allowed it, the venn diagram's spheres should be moving about the page and changing relative sizes and only ever occasionally intersecting. But that elusive intersection is our goal. Not everyone focuses on family when they really need to and that ends up being one of their regrets and regrets really suck the productive life out of you. Leave aside vague, warm fuzzy feelings that we all should be able to get everything out of all these separate parts of our life because underlying that is a belief that they are separate parts of our life. They needn't and shouldn't be.

Research into the longest-living and the happiest people on Earth shows that they manage to treat life as life and manage to spend the bulk of their time in that overlap. It has no separate parts that the majority of us modern, industrialised, western societies arbitrarily and abstractly segment our time into. That's counter-productive and unhealthy, whereas this book is about being productive and healthy, based on an interdependent and interwoven web of all these strands of our life where each strand supports the others. We work for those we love and we're enabled to be better at our work because of the reciprocated support. If we don't have that we, and they, suffer for it. I'll stress early and often throughout this book that I'm no tree-hugging bleeding-heart liberal hippy. There needs to be practical outcomes. There needs to be a point.

The point of life is work and the point of work is love and the point of love is life. You gotta make a buck but it's never for its own sake.

In my extensive research for this book, I read 100 books and a 100 research papers so you don't have to. Most people don't. Most people might skim a misleading headline from the online lifestyle section of the local newspaper once a day, with tips on how to stay bikini-ready during the calorie-laden festive season or how a once-absolute medical truth has been disproven or how a celebrity reveals their two secret techniques for looking younger, only one of which is Photoshop. I read a lot about how life spans have stretched from averaging in the late 20s in caveman times to the late 40s as recently as the early 19th century to about 80 today. But historical figures were skewed lower by child mortality rates. In Shakespeare's home town, Stratford-Upon-Avon's adult population between 1570 and 1630, one third of the men and one fifth of the women were over 60 years of age. Kids did not have a great track record of surviving and all those who died young drove down the averages. Those that did make it to adulthood then tended to keep on keeping on. Removing that child mortality factor, the life expectancy of a sixty year old white American male has only increased five years in the last 50 years. (I use white American males as the literature seems to think they're the most important. They're certainly the most advantaged.)

Jonathan Swift wrote, "Every man desires to live long but no man would be old." A 2005 poll by *USA Today* and *ABC Television* concluded that most people would be happy to live to 87. Their top concerns along the way were losing health and becoming unable to take care of themselves.

We want what's called 'compression of morbidity.' We want to keep on going until we don't. We want that imaginary line graph of our life, energy, health and purpose to keep on trucking until a dignified end, not tailing off from a mid-point and slumping for a miserable and intolerably long home stretch. Cancers, Diabetes, Heart disease and Lung disease will be what kills 9 out of 10 people in industrialised nations. And what's worse is that those types of causes of death inflict a long period of unproductive unhappiness prior to the end.

I'm not a doctor. More specifically, I'm not a doctor with a vested or financial interest in peddling to you my programme or diet or product that will keep you looking young or magically reverse the damage your choices up to this point have done to your body's systems. I'm a people engagement expert who teaches, writes and speaks to businesses. Personally, I did the research behind this book for purely selfish reasons. My father died when he was 45 and I was 2. I recently turned 47. He had some bad luck and made some poor choices. Using some of the online tools I'll show you in this book, I found that my 'real' age is 40 and, bad luck aside, I am likely to live to 99 in pretty good knick if I make some smarter choices.

To whatever extent those forecasts are accurate, they provoked and motivated me to extend my productive life. I don't know about 99 but it is realistic for me to add 10 years to whatever my baseline is. I love my work. I don't really consider it to be work in the usual pejorative sense we use the word. I have no intention of retiring when a Government says I should.

I plan to set an amazing example for my kids, not by living the 100%-sugar-&-fat-free life of a food-martyr but by blending my worlds of life, work and love and making smart, informed and moderate choices - because I want to, not because I'm made to feel that I'm supposed to. Although I will be cutting back sugar, sweeteners and refined white carbs to the max. More on that later.

I'd like to inspire others to do the same – starting with you right now.

2

Your Personal Systems:
One Size Does Not Fit All

83% of people living to 100 are female. Lads, this doesn't extrapolate to meaning that a gender reassignment procedure will boost your longevity. Beware of over-simplified recommendations based on stats. Correlation does not equal cause and effect. Throughout this book, I'll present a lot of research findings and stats. Some are inherently contradictory but I'll include some of those as it provides the context that there isn't one clear, obvious and common approach for all. However, there are a lot of overlapping and consistent findings. These form the basis of the twelve controls I'll expand on in Section 5.3.

What I'm providing is a toolbox, not an instruction manual. Tools are OK if you use them as they're supposed to be used. A hammer is a great tool for banging in nails. If you use it to brush your teeth, any damage done is not the fault of the hammer.

Get to know yourself. Nothing about health is one-size-fits-all and what I'll be suggesting in this book is a personalised approach, driven by yourself. That's why I'm calling the twelve tools 'Controls.'

One study of centenarians ranked their self-perceptions of what they thought helped them to stick around and to keep in relatively good condition doing so:

- Attitude,
- Healthy eating,
- Faith,
- Keeping active,
- Clean living,
- Family,
- Genetics.

Self reporting is interesting but they could well be wrong. And they are. The top factors are genetics, socialization, diet, and keeping physically active. And even then, those are sweeping generalisations. You need to know, given the cards you've been genetically dealt, how to play your hand.

Having just dissed averages and generalisations, they are useful indicators of the smartest behaviours to start with looking at in ourselves. Of those centenarians:

80% considered themselves to be optimistic but realistic,

78% never dieted in their entire lives (37% of girls currently in their teens have dieted and 14% of boys. Have you?),

100% recommended moderate portions and chewing your food,

<30% ever formally exercised but 100% were always "very active,"

75% never smoked,

0% had a criminal record.

That last one is interesting. Making good decisions and conscientiousness are highly correlated with longevity and good health. Committing crimes is incongruent with making good decisions and conscientiousness.

The usual throwaway advice given to those who want to improve their health (relax, eat veges, lose weight, get married) are lifesaving for some but neither effective or affordable for many. Mark Twain said, "We cannot reach old age by another man's road. My habits protect my life but they would assassinate you." Of course, he probably said that with a cigar between his teeth and his 4th glass of bourbon in his hand so let's not focus too much on Twain, although he did live to 75.

A consistent theme throughout this book is inter-connectedness – a systems approach. Certainly, when you get to the sections on our bodies and how our physical systems work (or don't), this becomes incredibly evident. But it's also true of the interconnectedness of our physical, mental and social dimensions.

This next piece of research might be more of a laugh than anything factually helpful but it is a conversation starter. I use it when MCing conferences to get a buzz going and the noise and enthusiasm levels up amongst the audience.

John Manning studied the relationship between our finger lengths and certain health outcomes. Look at the photo below of my hand and how I've marked the difference in length between my ring finger (4D) and my index finger (2D.) Check out your own 4D:2D ratio. They've been the same your whole life and they're not going to change. It's supposed that their relative lengths are a consequence of exposure to differing levels of testosterone in the womb as a foetus.

So what? Manning's study of Liverpool heart attack victims' fingers found a high ratio (like mine) has a correlation with lower heart attack risk. It's good for sport. It's bad for depression. It's terrible for autism. Manning himself describes his findings as, "Persuasive but not yet definitive." Why am I even bothering to finish this paragraph?

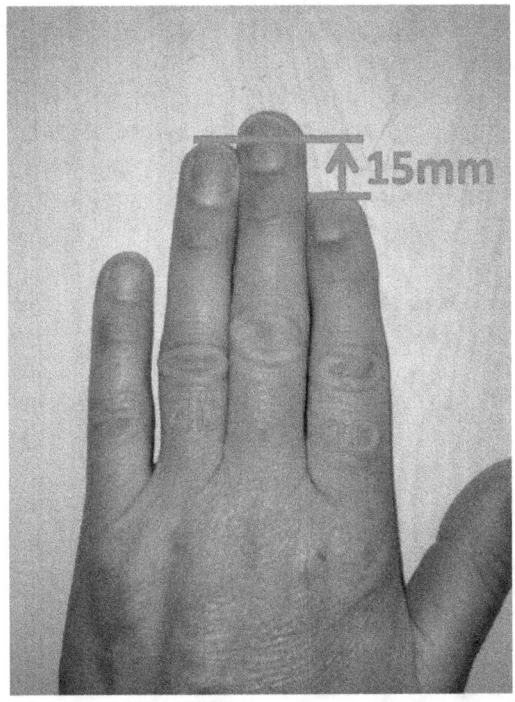

You're too busy trying to stretch your fingers or finding a friend to check out their fingers before you tell them why...

More recent research by the University of Florida into digit ratio using mice proved conclusively that relative digit length is indeed governed by prenatal exposure to the sex hormones testosterone and oestrogen. (I've never seen mice give other mice 'the finger' but it would seem that they are indeed capable. Their digit relativity is similar to humans.) The researchers were Martin Cohn and Zhenghui Zheng. Cohn commented, "When he came back with the initial results, I was blown away. We looked at each others' hands, then got busy planning the next experiment."

Your finger lengths and the 2D:4D activity are a memorable example of something that might be affecting your chances but over which you have no control. This book will offer broad menus of things you _**can** do_ to improve the quality and quantity of your life, extend the productive period of your life and encourage those you love to do so too. But what you actually end up doing must be highly personalised, as we're all very different.

I got quite worried reading some stats about how some quite mainstream and 'popular' meds just don't work for some people and the medical establishment doesn't know why not. We're that different. Even our gut microbes are different. Later in this book, you'll read how some futurists predict that there will be probiotic cafes where we can all pop in for a smoothie with personalised gut bacteria. I'll be making my bacteria smoothie a takeaway, as keeping moving is one of the twelve controls I'm using much more since I did the research for this book. I'm typing this right now whilst standing up.

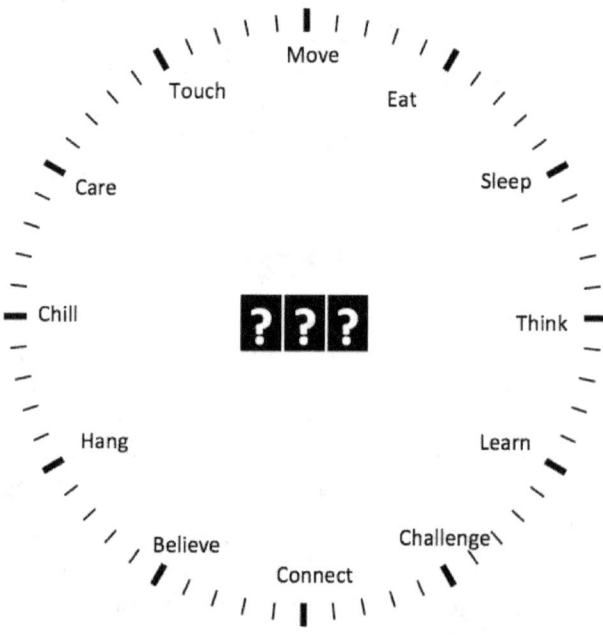

More about those twelve controls and probiotic smoothies later. First, let's give ourselves some context by looking at how we got to where we are today when it comes to our attitudes on aging, health and productivity.

3

The History and Future of Not Dying

For the largest part of human history, life was brutish and short. Now, in my country New Zealand, depending on your gender and race, you can expect to live to close to eighty. How well you live is mostly up to you.

Humans have had three traditional approaches to dealing with the prospect of death:

1. Some form of religious 'hereafter' or reincarnation option,

2. Creating some lasting contribution or legacy that will exist even once you do not,

3. Trying not to die.

If you're not a pushy jerk or hate-mongering fundamentalist, rightly or wrongly (wrongly), option 1 might make you feel better and can actually generate longevity-enhancing health benefits, as I'll discuss later. Option 2 is a pretty good idea on its own merits and, it too, might bolster your sense of purpose and thus drive some physiological benefits for you personally beyond the contribution you're making to others. This book will look at all three options but primarily the third, although I'll expand "trying not to die" to a more positive, realistic and measurable, "living 10 more quality and productive years." And to make it not all about you, I'll include how you can help those you love extend their 'healthy life expectancy' too.

Checking back into various religious and cultural tales, some figures could really crank out the living back in the day. Methuselah supposedly got to 969 years of age. (He knew Adam and Eve but didn't make even a cameo on Noah's ark.) Mesopotamia's reign of 10 kings totalled 432,000 years which meant they each averaged 43,200 years. Chinese monarchs had a few reigns around 18,000 years. I presume these are the 'good old days' to which people often refer?

In Greek mythology, Achilles' mum Thetis dipped him as a baby in the river Styx making him invulnerable, except for his heel. That heel ultimately led to his death in the Trojan War. His Mum should've double-dipped him, except he was a Demi-God, not a corn chip.

Water features heavily in the history of longevity and such. The Garden of Eden had four rivers leading out from a central spring. Various 'Fountain of Youth' myths over the millennia work that missing and mysterious H2O into their symbolism and mythology.

Stories abound of mythical rejuvenating potions like that of Medea The Enchantress that contained roots, seeds, flowers, stag liver and werewolf entrails. If you were able to get possession of a werewolf's entrails, chances are, you were in serious need of some rejuvenation. Plus, who wouldn't believe someone whose job title contained the word "Enchantress"?

Comedian Heath Franklin created the larger-than-life-but-based-on-real-life character 'Chopper.' Outfitted in sunglasses, tatts and toughness, one of my favourite lines from him to modern metrosexual men is, "Drink a cup of concrete and harden the @#$% up." Chopper is figuratively a Stoic. The original Stoics were philosophers in the third century BC. Seneca wrote 'De Brevitate Vitae' (The Shortness Of Life) which included this quote, "In practice, people only live a tiny part of their lives. Why should we ask nature for more when we are already incapable of taking advantage of what it has already given us?" Seneca later killed himself so whilst he was literally a Stoic, he wasn't in practice particularly stoic.

Attila the Hun legendarily died at the age of 124, not in the heat of battle but during sex with his newest and youngest wife. Kind of a glass-half-full deal that one.

English Friar Roger Bacon (1220-1292) recommended a diet of meat, egg yolks, red wine and boiled vipers. Typically English – boiling their vipers. Probably you'd be better off stir-frying them in an olive oil.

Nostradamus (1503-1566) the famed predictor of the future wrote that the best way to extend your life was to move from place to place in alignment with the shifts in astrological elements. So, not only was he a shonky Astrologer, it seems likely that he was a shonky real estate agent as well.

Sir Francis Bacon (1561-1626), in addition to being Lord Chancellor, Attorney General and maybe being the real writer of Shakespeare's better works is also credited with developing what we now call The Scientific Method. (Hypothesis, Experiment, Observe, Repeat.) So, to a degree, without him, we wouldn't today enjoy the TV show 'The Big Bang Theory.' His advice was for trapping the life force within the body by rubbing the body with old butter after cold baths. He also recommended opium and powdered gold. Hey, we've all been there after a hard night on the opium and powdered gold, waking up covered in cold butter think, "Wow, I hope I can spend the next 150 years like this." I think the period Bacon lived in was known as 'The Enlightenment'?

Today's dogma is tomorrow's heresy. Eggs are bad. Eggs are good. Different parts of eggs are different. Aargh!

The longest human lifespan verified and certified was the French woman Jeanne Louise Calment who made a respectable innings of 122. (1875-1997.) Something of an Enchantress herself, she was feisty, once claiming, "I've never had but one wrinkle and I'm sitting on it."

The over-riding theme I've picked up from my reading of the many doctors, gerontologists and futurists who are confident that one day soon technology will invent or discover the magic bullet to prevent or reverse aging is that it is going to happen and our priority in the meantime is to keep breathing until it does. Be it splicing chromosomes, nanobots cleaning us out at a cellular level or some hormonal potion, they think that, like global warming, there'll be a solution prompted by economic forces driving technological advances. I don't buy that myself but I will take up their 'keep breathing' advice.

Cryogenic facilities exist for those with money and wishful thinking to preserve their bodies after death so they might be rejuvenated once technology catches up with their imaginations. Alcor in Scotsdale, Arizona and the Cryonics Institute in Clinton, Michigan will take your money and write you a receipt, although where you're going, you don't need receipts.

Don't laugh at the promises of technology. Already Google can predict outbreaks of illnesses before centres for disease control. If a bunch of people all start Googling symptoms at the same time in the same place, Google knows that. They could tell the authorities or invest in shares in vaccine companies.

The only proven scientific intervention that prolongs longevity is calorie reduction. The body's systems want to exist long enough to breed and to give the offspring as much chance to survive as possible. Times of famine are not great for that so the body tunes itself to last longer, waiting for what it perceives as the famine time to pass. Tests done with rats showed this was possible but there were downsides. Reproductive development was delayed or stunted. Those released in the wild perished as their bodies sacrificed hardiness for longevity – a high price to pay. Just living longer is not what people want. (No one asked the rats.)

The first studies into the effects on rats of calorie restriction took place during the great depression. Society wondered if people going hungry could bounce back from periods of hunger without serious or significant long-term effects. Rats that normally could expect to live to 600 days got up to 870 days.

Scientists have also generated plasticity in the aging of fruit flies through selective breeding, effectively accelerating evolution in a lab. Good news for a species that has one day to get laid.

Beware of scientific breakthrough headlines in the media. 'The Economist' wrote in 2013, "Last year researchers at one biotech firm, Amgen, found they could reproduce just six of 53 landmark studies in cancer research. Earlier, a group at Bayer, a drug company, managed to repeat just a quarter of 67 similarly important papers. The obligation to publish or perish has come to rule over academic life. Careerism also encourages exaggeration and the cherry-picking of results. The most striking findings have the greatest chance of making it onto the page. If they touch on drinking wine, going senile or letting children play video games, they may well command the front pages of newspapers too. Conversely, failures to prove a hypothesis are rarely even offered for publication, let alone accepted. Negative results now account for only 14% of published papers, down from 30% in 1990."

Remember Sir Francis Bacon and the scientific method? After the hypothesis and the experiment, there is testing and observing to prove or disprove the hypothesis, then a conclusion. The critical next step is replication. Experiments need to be able to be replicated. The Economist article suggests that this keystone of scientific advancement is suffering due to the same economic forces driving our increased consumption of poor food and increased participation in unhealthy inactivity.

If there could be a happy marriage of science and the commercial imperative for profit, maybe Google can find it. In September 2013, Google announced the launch of *Calico*, a new company that will focus on health and well-being, in particular the challenge of aging and associated diseases. Check out the movies "Prometheus' and 'Wolverine 2' for a couple of possible outcomes for when billionaire company owners start projects so they can live forever.

There have been genuine surges in lifespan and healthspan over time due to collective jumps in societies' success in food production and distribution, education, hygiene and welfare. I believe the next big surge will be due to technology enabling us all to have a much more individualised and informed ability to guide our lifestyle choices. The definite trend over recorded human history regarding longevity and wellness is a decline of the reliance on Gods and magic and increasingly we're accepting that, collectively and individually, we need to rely more upon our own choices. If it's meant to be, it's up to me, or more accurately, <u>you</u>.

4

Prolonging Personal Productivity

"The longer I live, the more beautiful life is." – Frank Lloyd Wright

My focus in this book is to enable us to add productive and meaningful years to our lives when we need them, not tagging on a few more feeble ones at the end. It's a hot topic of great interest as economists, unions and politicians around the world argue about raising the age of eligibility for Government retirement plans and such.

There are a lot of other motivations, judging by the books in the library around the subject of longevity and wellness. Many are targeting people:

- Not wanting to look old because they think that would be a bad thing,

- Whose bodies and minds are starting to break down and they'd like some miraculous trick to turn back the clock,

- Who think they're the wrong shape / size / weight.

The primacy of youthfulness is a recent product of western advertisers since the 1950s. Those who were actually youths in the 1950s are now greying baby boomers smashing into the brick wall of retirement age.

By the year 2050, a fifth of humanity will be over 60 years of age. In Europe, it'll be 37%. In the ten years to 2009, demand for traditional facelifts fell by 23%. In the same period, demand for lazer skin resurfacing rose 154% and demand for botox treatment rose 504%. These numbers would raise eyebrows if, indeed, your botoxed eyebrows were still capable of being raised.

The first writings that distinguished a period of childhood occurred in the 15th century. The term 'teenager' wasn't popularised until the 1940s. The term 'ageism' was first used in 1968. Gradually we're adding to the age stages we're supposed to experience. Shakespeare had his seven ages of man and that didn't include teenagers which, given that Romeo and Juliet were thirteen, may not be surprising.

We're experiencing the benefits of technological augmentation. We've had spectacles for centuries. Hearing aids are ever-improving. Teeth are not what they used to be. The internet's apps and information are available to assist. My personal favourite is the promise of nanotechnology – little robots at a cellular level that they'll inject into us to sort out the crappy molecules. Nothing to worry about - brought to you by the same people who brought us photocopiers that never screw up.

Walt Disney said of any quest for success, "Observe what the masses do then do the opposite." Beware the latest crazes for staying young and cheating death. Robert Park's *Quackwatch* has a helpful list of criteria that are a giveaway as to the likelihood of the fad being fraudulent:

1.   The discoverer pitches the claim direct to the media,

2.   The discoverer says a powerful establishment is trying to suppress their work,

3.   The scientific effect involved is always at the very limit of detection,

4.   Evidence is anecdotal,

5.   The discoverer says a belief is credible because it has endured for centuries,

6.   The discoverer has worked in isolation,

7. The discoverer must propose new laws of nature to explain an observation.

That said, the future will hold amazing advances – eventually. It's not the big, magic bullet advances that will help as much as many small changes we each choose to make. And we know what they are today and do not need to wait for someone in a white lab coat carrying the modern equivalent of a clipboard to tell us. It might be that in ten years time, there'll be a chain of cafes as successful as StarBucks is today, except it won't sell coffees, they'll be probiotic cafes to amp up our gut microbes.

More reasonable and real-world-based scientists chase the world's pockets of oldsters determined to glean secrets from those who have lived the longest. Usually they're in remote locations and have been chasing goats up steep hillsides their entire lives. (The oldsters, not the scientists.) The best of these and highly recommended is Dan Buettner's 'Blue Zones.'

He identified four locations with disproportionate numbers of centenarians – Okinawa in Japan, Nicoya in Costa Rica, Loma Linda in California, and Barbagia in Sardinia. From these folk, he distilled nine tips:

- Move,
- Eat til you're not hungry,
- Plant slant,
- Grapes of life,
- Purpose now!,
- Down shift,
- Belong,
- Loved ones first,
- Right tribe.

For a fun conversation starter at dinner parties, I suggest the Blue Zones Vitality Quiz at

http://apps.bluezones.com/vitality/. If you answer the questions as honestly as you can, it'll give you an estimate of how long you might expect to live. Then, more usefully, it'll provide a few behaviour changes and a revised age goal if you follow their advice. Right or wrong, it's a clever tool to provoke action and highlight individual issues. It's free and you don't get spammed afterwards.

The New England Centenarian Study found a few common behaviours amongst the longer living people they assessed:

1. Eat and drink in moderation,

2. Stay in touch with friends and make new friends,

3. Optimism (Although this is a result of living longer, not the cause),

4. A sense of humour,

5. Have multiple interests,

6. Deliberately challenge their brains,

7. Engaged in a life purpose.

A 2003 study of centenarians by the Ohio University School of Medicine confirmed that there is more than one way to live a long and healthy life. They pre-supposed that centenarians had managed to avoid life-threatening illnesses or significantly delayed them. What they found was gender differences and three categories of centenarian when it came to age-associated diseases: Escapers, Delayers and Survivors.

	Male	*female*
Survivors	24%	43%
Delayers	44%	42%
Escapers	32%	15%

When examining only the most lethal diseases of the elderly population, heart disease, non-skin cancer and stroke, they found that 87% of male and 83% of female subjects delayed or escaped these diseases.

I conclude from this that, while it is possible to survive, it'd be better to not have to. Delaying is preferable. Escaping is best. It's all about positively influencing your odds.

Okinawa crops up in many references as a Mecca of longevity and, yes, it has a disproportionately high ratio of people living to at least 100. But, there is a context that make the causes of that longevity even more stark. After World War II, the Americans established a naval base there. It's big. It's a significant employer and generates a lot of local economic activity and cultural influence. And along with all that economic activity and cultural influence came the Westernised diet.

Wiki Travel says of Okinawa, "Aficionados of American fast food may find Okinawa to be a curious treat, as many American restaurants popped up here to serve the US military long before they made it to the mainland. Most prominent is the presence of A&W outlets serving hamburgers and root beer (with free refills, even), available practically nowhere else in Japan. Foremost ice cream (under the "Blue Seal" brand) is also common. Several hybrid Okinawan-American dishes, most of which seem to employ copious quantities of Spam, are widely available. The *Nuuyaru burger* (ぬーやるバーガー), a speciality of local fast food chain Jef is gōyā champurū, cheese and a slice of Spam in a bun. Appropriately enough, the name is an Okinawan pun that translates roughly as "What on earth is this?"

The generations following this influx has the same rate of health related disorders such as diabetes and heart disease as the U.S.

What matters are the quality of the relationships we form and the parenting we provide. I don't know if it's relevant but

Dan Buettner, author of Blue Zones, is married to 80s super model Cheryl Tiegs.

Doctor David Agus in his book 'The End Of Illness' suggests taking a regular personal health inventory and provides a long long list of questions to ask yourself. I got bored after the 9th item and I suspect I would be fairly typical. The key point is to be on the alert for changes. Only you know what your 'normal' is and any prolonged deviations from your 'normal' need checking out. Some of his checklist questions were:

- Overall, how are you feeling? Is there a trend / pattern?

- How are your energy levels?

- How regular is your schedule?

- How's your breathing?

- Has your ability to exercise changed?

- Has your walk changed?

- Are you experiencing any new or changed sensations?

- Anything weird going on with your skin?

- Are you having a lot of bad hair days?

I've paraphrased some of the above questions but I've definitely noticed that I get bad hair days immediately before I ever come down with anything. It's my own personal little health barometer. One day my hair went grey and then I became a father. (Actually, that might have been the other way around.)

I've read the books and by-and-large, it's not complicated to improve your odds of keeping yourself healthy and productive, and slowing aging's decline of your body's systems. It's not a lot of secrets either. Yet, most people with knowledge won't make any changes. I'll provide some techniques to help you increase your odds of making changes and making them stick a bit later as well. But most people reveal in their behaviour that they choose not to keep themselves healthy and productive, nor slow aging's decline of their body's systems. They choose to eat the pie.

You'll be fine but not most people. It's a running gag in the sitcom 'The Big Bang Theory' that Penny's *check engine light* is always on yet she never checks the engine. It's funny because it's relatable and typical behaviour. But do you imagine if you got a warning to make a change or you would die, that you would? You probably think you would. You might think that everyone would choose life. We can all surmise and hypothesise but what really reveals us is our behaviour when such scenarios get real. Here are some stats from people who have had a heart attack or kidney failure, events that used to be a death sentence and, even today, are a real wake-up call warning shot across the bow. How many of these people who survive and get a second chance actually comply with their recommended life saving treatment? Surely, it's 100%? Nope. Non-compliance means smoking, breaking diet, failing to take meds, missing appointments and discontinuing monitoring.

Non-Compliance After Organ Transplant:

- Kidney – 20-50%
- Heart – 30%

So, most people don't have whatever they need in their life to make them want to live well and more, even when they get a slap in the face to do so. In 2013, actress Angelina Jolie received much attention when, after DNA tests showed that there was a very high statistical likelihood of her developing breast cancer, she opted for pre-emptive mastectomy surgery. That was a courageous decision even with evidence that she must have considered overwhelming. But what if you had similar data and the solution wasn't radical invasive surgery but simply eating better every day?

I have a colleague in my circle of performing acquaintances who has been diagnosed with a disease that is a precursor to colon cancer. It's not a 'maybe'; If you get this precursor, there is a 100% chance you will get colon cancer. That is one of the more awful cancers both in its mortality rates and in the consequences of dealing with its aftermath if you survive. The only variable at debate is the timing. But it will happen.

To me, it seems that the precursor condition is a blessing – a warning sign before it's too late. Not only can colon cancer be avoided if behaviour changes are implemented but even the precursor condition can be cured. I have things to accomplish with my life yet and I want to see my kids grow up. All these and other things motivate me to want to live and do what it takes. But, that's me.

The behaviour changes are not permanent invasive surgery. They're just behaviour changes – diet and exercise. This person is a vegetarian but has a super-high cholesterol and sugar diet with minimal actual vegetables, plus a super-inactive lifestyle. In short, he is not changing his behaviour. He knows at a reasoned and conscious level what the inevitable consequences will be. He's still not changing.

I do not understand this, nor do I understand those non-compliant heart-attack survivors. I can't make them change. Their doctors can't make them change. Their mothers can't.

That's why this is personal and specific. There is no one right way. It has to begin with you *wanting* to live longer and better before it becomes a desperate need or a foregone conclusion. And your reason needs to be effective and enduringly motivating for you.

The rest of this book is in three parts: Live, Work and Love. The foundation of this structure is that we want to stay alive and healthy to work. I use the term 'work' in a broad sense – to be creative, to have purpose, to make a contribution, as well as the run-of-the-mill earning money. And that work is for a reason – we do it for those we love. And, in turn, we are better enabled to live and work, because of those we love. It's all interconnected and unique to you.

So, away you go. Let me give you some control. Or, to be more precise, twelve controls.

5

LIVE

"The idea is to die young as late as possible." – Ashley Montague

The systems in your body typically begin to decline at about age twenty. They're all inter-related and inter-dependent. The primary systems are your heart (circulatory), lungs (respiratory) and brain (nervous system.) The secondary systems are your immune, digestive, endocrine (hormones) and musculo-skeletal. Danish studies on separated identical twins, indicate that how long you live and how well your systems keep operating is due to 30% genetic luck and 70% lifestyle choices.

70%! That's a lot of control you have. Follow the tips. Use the controls. Or don't. Just don't complain when you're dead.

5.1

Causes of Aging / Physical and Mental Deterioration

Seven out of ten Americans would prefer to die at home on their terms. Seven out of ten Americans actually die invalided and intubated in an institution.

In 2013, The Washington Post reported on a study which was conducted by scientists from the University of Southern California, Harvard University, Columbia University, the University of Illinois at Chicago and other institutions.

"When we treat someone with cancer, or heart disease, or stroke, we are treating a manifestation or by-product of biological aging -- the underlying process marches on unaltered by this approach to disease," said Jay Olshansky, a professor at the University of Illinois School of Public Health in Chicago and a co-author of the study.

"This means that even if we succeed for a time in extending life by treating a disease, either that disease or another will emerge with time....Slowing aging alters the risk of all diseases simultaneously by attacking the origins of all of the things that go wrong with us as we grow older."

Are aging and death inevitable to prevent the over-crowding and resource depletion of our planet? Time happens and stuff happens. Through bad luck and poor choices, you will experience some or all of the following in combination. These age you in a biological sense:

- Inflammation (Chronic not acute.)
- Oxidative Stress (Free radicals looking for electrons)
- Glycation (Tangled sugar & protein molecules)
- Methylation (DNA's blueprint function gets messed up.)
- Immunity impairment

Regardless of what's going in with your biological aging, the three factors driving how old you look are:

- Obesity,
- Smoking,
- Over-stressing.

I'll go into much more detail later on but, broadly, here are some behaviour choices available to you to mitigate each of the aging processes:

Inflammation

Be in a healthy weight range

- Move!
- Eat good fats
- Eat garlic

Oxidation

- Eat the rainbow
- Moderate exercise

Glycation

- Don't eat anything ending in "...ose" (Sugars)
- Eat blueberries

Methylation

- Eat eggs
- Eat seeds
- Check your meds

Immunity

- Wash your hands
- Get vaccinated
- Don't smoke
- Don't overuse antibiotics

On top of these and other possible causes of aging, is the big one – built-in obsolescence. Our DNA blueprint is inherently 'on the clock' with cells having a finite number of reproductions programmed in. This finite number of divisions of cells is known as the 'Hayflick Limit.'

In the mid 60s, Leonard Hayflick found that cells go through three phases. The first is rapid, healthy cell division. In the second phase, mitosis slows. In the third stage, senescence, cells stop dividing entirely. They remain alive for a time after they stop dividing, but sometime after cellular division ends, cells do a particularly disturbing thing: Essentially, they commit suicide. Once a cell reaches the end of its life span, it undergoes a programmed cellular death called apoptosis. Even freezing then thawing cells made no difference. They 'remembered' where they were in their countdown. We have a molecular clock that's winding down from the instant we're born. The question is – can we re-wind that clock? Normal human cells have a limited capacity for replication and, as yet, we don't have the technology to tweak that limitation.

Telomeres are our biological hourglass. At both ends of every chromosome are 'tails', sequences of DNA that are not

31

like other genetic material. You know that roll of paper in cash registers onto which receipts are printed? When it is nearing its end and needs to be replaced, a pink stripe appears. Telomeres are like the pink stripe indicating the nearing end of our chromosomes. They might better be described as like aglets. Aglets are the plastic tips at the ends of our shoelaces that prevent our shoelaces from getting frayed. Once that aglet goes, that shoelace is done for. Some scientists are investigating if the enzyme Telomerase might have the potential to rejuvenate human cells. However Telomerase is the same thing that helps cancer cells become so dominant. So, it's probably good for a back page article in MindFood magazine but may be just a flash of false hope in the pan. It seems unlikely that there will ever be one single thing, one silver anti-aging bullet. What's necessary to mitigate aging (an issue of systems decline) is a systemic approach – multiple strategies, not a single pill or superfood or positive thought programme. That said, Telomeres research won the Nobel Prize for medicine in 2009 and those researchers offer a lot of good advice.

One of the reviewers of their book described it as, "Chicken soup for the cells." Ironic, given that chicken soup would have way too much salt.

They offer a range of decent dietary and exercise advice, and promote meditation. But, they do massively stress the need to spend money on and consume a long list of expensive supplements:

- Omega-3 fish oil

- Acetyl-L-Carnitine

- Berry-derived anthocyanidins (Elderberries)

- N-Acetylcysteine

- 'Super' multivitamins

- CoQ10

- L-Carnosine

- Phosphatidylserine

- Alpha-lipoic acid

- TA-65 ($US2200-8000 per year)

The U.S Federal Drug Administration won't fund TA-65 and it can only be marketed as a 'supplement' which means it can't make any health or curative claims. The list above is a long list, won't be cheap and, personally, I wouldn't be happy putting so many pills into my body that I rattled when I walked.

Cholesterol gets a bad rap even now but our bodies produce it naturally and it's not the cholesterol per se that is the problem. Once it gets oxidized, then it's a problem.

What has been happening in recent decades that drives these diseases and decline when the Western world is so affluent? The answer is the affluence itself.

% Food $ Spent Away From Home

% Calories Eaten Away From Home

	% Food $ Spent Away From Home	**% Calories Eaten Away From Home**
1973	25%	18%
1986	35%	27%
1995	40%	34%

A 2001 study of 5000 people by the University of Minnesota found the following about the association between fast-food and overall consumption. (A sedentary male aged 31-50 averages a daily need of 2200 calories.):

Ave Fast Food Meals a Week	Avg Daily Calorie Intake
1-2	2192
3+	2753

A study of 5000 people and their fast food purchasing habits by Otago University found:

- Fish 'n' chips have been overtaken by sugar and refined carb laden bread-based foods such as pizza, burgers and sandwiches,

- Nearly 1/3 of New Zealanders report eating fast food on any one day,

- 19 to 30-year-olds eat the most fast food,

- Maori eat more fast food than NZ European and Pacific peoples,

- People in households of four or more eat more fast food,

- Single people eat more fast food than couples,

- People in cities are more likely to eat fast food,

- People with tertiary qualifications and higher incomes are more likely to eat at restaurants,

- Men are more likely than women to eat fast food,

- 14 per cent eat in a restaurant or cafe on any one day,

- Fast food makes up about nine per cent of our calories.

The causes of our aging and deterioration in an era of unprecedented longevity are what we're eating and what we're doing. Or, more accurately, what we're *not* doing. How's that working out for us?

5.2

Consequences of Aging / Physical and Mental Deterioration

*"You can't help getting older but you
don't have to get old." – George Burns*

David Katz in his book 'Disease-Proof' writes of a measurement called HALE (Healthy Life Expectancy.) This is much more useful for what we're trying to achieve with this book than just life expectancy. Living a long time is no great prize if you're in terrible shape, unhappy and unproductive. In 2010 in the U.S., the HALE for men was 65.0 years and for women it was 63.4 years. That left a gap of 13 years of **un**healthy life expectancy. Ouch! Let's you and me try to minimise that number.

As a young child, I would walk past my mum when she was on the phone with her best friend. One would relate her latest ailment then the other would top it with her latest ailment. Not to be outdone, each would ratchet up the ailment count in turn. It was like a game of high-stakes health poker – a game where, even if you win, you lose.

Getting old and wearing out isn't just a visual thing, nor one of getting ill. Just maintaining a modern existence becomes more effortful. Liberty Mutual Insurance runs a programme where they suit people up in gear that emulates the physical effects of driving for an average 80 year-old. The suit and bracing limit or slow body movements, diminish vision and distort posture. They then send participants out to a car on a closed track to perform various standard driving exercises with cones and a stopwatch. Obviously performance is substandard with many participants reporting how difficult they found it just getting to the car, getting in and buckling up.

Most obviously, the effects of aging are the visual ones of grey hair, balding, wrinkles, and getting flabby. A 1988 study by David Weeks pointed at the primary drivers of maintaining a youthful appearance being:

1. Genetic luck,

2. Exercise,

3. Sex.

A conversation starter (or stopper) if nothing else.

Even if science comes up with ways of making us physically immortal, statisticians have found that given human behaviour and luck, we would each likely encounter a fatal accident on average every 1200 years. Insurance adverts will be very different in the future. A long life may not be desirable if your friends and family are gone and you have nothing of substance to do or be in your extra years.

In New Zealand, health insurer Southern Cross has listed the top five surgical claims for different age groups, showing what men and women claim for. Crack open your diaries and book ahead. If you don't start taking better preventative care of yourself, the following is what you have to look forward to:

Top procedures* claimed for in 2012, ranked by age

Top 5 procedures, 20-29 age band

- Women: Removal of teeth, endometriosis surgery, freeing abdominal adhesions, ovarian cystectomy, excision skin lesion.

- Men: Removal of teeth, excision skin lesion, septoplasty, hernia repair, colonoscopy.

Top 5 procedures, 30-39

- Women: Endometriosis surgery, hysterectomy, excision skin lesion, cholecystectomy, removal of teeth.

- Men: Removal of teeth, colonoscopy, excision skin lesion, hernia repair, septoplasty.

Top 5 procedures, 40-49

- Women: Hysterectomy, hysteroscopy, excision skin lesion, colonoscopy, endometriosis surgery.

- Men: Colonoscopy, excision skin lesion, hip replacement, hernia repair, coronary angioplasty.

Top 5 procedures, 50-59

- Women: Colonoscopy, hysterectomy, hip replacement, excision skin lesion, knee replacement.

- Men: Hip replacement, colonoscopy, excision skin lesion, coronary angioplasty, hernia repair.

Top 5 procedures, 60-69

- Women: Knee replacement, hip replacement, colonoscopy, cataract, excision skin lesion.

- Men: Knee replacement, hip replacement, excision skin lesion, coronary angioplasty, colonoscopy.

Top 5 procedures, 70 plus

- Women: Cataract, hip replacement, knee replacement, excision skin lesion, colonoscopy.

- Men: Knee replacement, cataract, hip replacement, excision skin lesion, coronary angioplasty.

*Of course, any particularly dramatic emergency procedures will get done in the public health system and so aren't listed here...

You probably want to avoid hospitals generally anyway. That's where sick people congregate. They do great work but if you want to contract an antibiotic resistant superbug, that'd be a place to start. 'Medical Tourism' is a thing these days. Developing nations with socialised health systems perform procedures for fee paying overseas visitors. The country's health system gets an injection of funds and the tourists get much cheaper medical interventions. A friend of mine got major dentistry done in Thailand. Michelle Duff in stuff.co.nz reported about a New Zealander who got one of those superbugs in Vietnam. The antibiotic age is barely a century old and already experts are talking of a 'Post-Antibiotic Age.' Earlier this year, British chief medical officer Sally Davies described resistance to antibiotics as a "catastrophic global threat" that should be ranked alongside terrorism. Go easy on the antibiotics and do what you can to stay as healthy as you can for as long as you can.

Professor Chris Maher, the Director of the Musculoskeletal Division at the George Institute for Global Health says, "At any point in time, 25-30 per cent of the population will have back pain and up to 80 per cent of people will have back pain at some time in their life." When it comes to back pain, the Sydney Morning Herald cites Maher as saying that a simple analgesic such as paracetamol is considered the best first option. However, the most common medications recommended or prescribed were non-steroidal anti-inflammatories (37 per cent), followed by opioids (20 per cent), with paracetamol coming in last (18 per cent). Fewer than one in five patients received paracetamol. The best medicine in most cases of non-specific back pain is to keep moving and take aspirin. More often, you'll get told to rest up and pop pills.

Heart disease is responsible for about 40% of all U.S. deaths. 11% of Americans consider themselves to be 'very overweight.' The Centre for Disease Control and Prevention states that the figure is actually 68%. So, there is a gap between perception and reality, leading to inaction which gives the U.S. the health track record it has, despite spending more on health per capita than any other nation on Earth.

The USA spends 17.8% of GDP on healthcare. That's four times what they spend on defence. That surprised me. More than half of that health spending is spent on people in the last two years of their life.

There's a tradition amongst parents to chart the heights of their children as they grow, usually on a wall or the back of a closet door. They shouldn't have to live in a lifestyle of our making where we chart their *widths*.

5.3

The 12 Controls

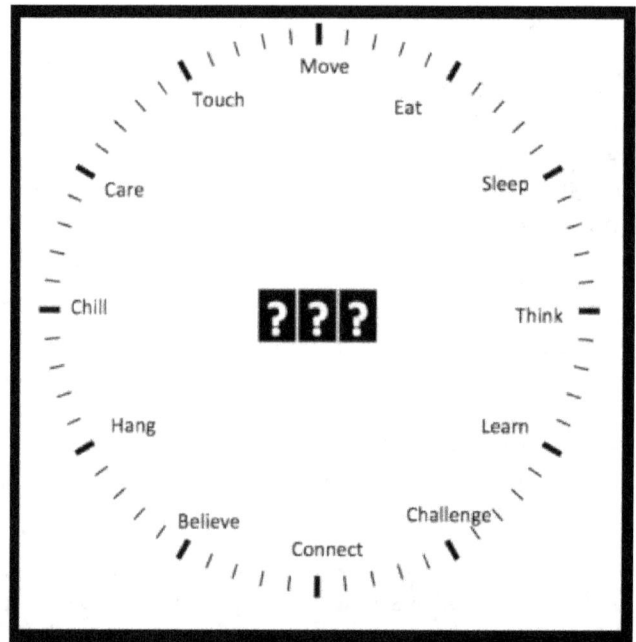

A lot of Doctors release books. Some of them are a bit dodgy and many contradict other Doctors. Some contradict themselves. On top of all that advice, you can choose from advisors describing themselves as 'Medical Intuitives' and others who use the word 'Aura' way too much. (ie more than zero.) I found one who suggested that, subconsciously, we all know what food is best for us and what is harmful. Initially this sounded like it had potential and was in line with my favoured personalised approach to food, physiology and the brain. So, I was a little disappointed when the next bit of advice was to hold a pendulum over the food and the sway would indicated whether or not we should eat it.

I found one book that listed page-by-page various influencers on your health and life spans, with debits and credits for each. All this is highly generalised and the numbers would obviously vary given individuals, genetics and the inter-relationship between factors. I was in a supermarket queue behind an older gentleman (older than me, so old) and he was buying coleslaw. He declined the free dressing that came with it due to its fat content. He then proceeded to ask for 2 packets of cigarettes. You're going to have to eat a mountain of low-fat coleslaw to offset smoking buddy. Unless he was smoking the coleslaw? Old trick from the Great Depression. Explains his rejecting the dressing.

Also, I disagree with some of the factors based on other research I've found. For example, +9 for happiness is wrong. Happiness is a consequence of a long and happy life, not a cause of it. This is a 'Log cabin' fallacy. People look at log cabins that still exist today and assume people back in the good old days were really good at making log cabins. They weren't. They were terrible but the good ones survived and remain still. They're the ones we observe, fuelling our fallacy. We don't see the crappy ones. It's the same with happiness and old people.

The Sovereign Wellbeing Index put out by AUT University looked at New Zealand wellbeing as part of a global study with 23 nations. Their analysis of the top 25% - those with what they called 'super-wellbeing' found the following factors driving their great lives:

- Connecting,
- Giving,
- Taking notice,
- Keeping learning,
- Being active,

- Non smoking,

- Exercise,

- Healthier diets,

- Higher income,

- Healthier weight.

Having read that and so much other research, when it comes to living, I'm recommending twelve controls. Partly, this is so I can create a visual model that looks like a combination clock, speedometer and odometer. The twelve fall into three distinct categories: Physical, Mental and Social – all inter-related.

Let's get physical.

5.3.1

Physical

"Nothing in excess." – Temple of Apollo, Delphi

At the time of writing, there is a series of amusing TV adverts promoting medical check-ups for men. Over 6000 men in New Zealand die from heart disease or diabetes-related disease each year. I applaud the adverts, the effort and the intention. It is all a bit late though, as much of the damage has been done by the time people hit their 40s. There is a prevalent mindset that we can keep up our pie-munching, cola-slurping, couch-denting lifestyles and then we can sort it out later. The 6000 deaths are the tip of an iceberg of illness, decline, unhappiness and unproductiveness.

Diabetes is, in itself, pretty bad but it can also cause or contribute to other conditions, making them worse in conjunction with the Diabetes, such as sleep apnea, blindness and cardiovascular disease. Very rarely do people just have Diabetes and if they do, it won't be for long. It is not even a condition of aging. 44% of diabetes-related deaths in Australia in 2013 occurred in people under the age of 60.

My own local medical centre makes an effort at preventive healthcare. My last birthday clicked over on their database and I automatically received a letter advising me that I had won... free blood and urine tests. I took the tests and got a glowing report on my lack of potential heart disease. I was halfway out of my chair about to depart the room when they told me to sit back down. I got a figurative slap across the face when it came to the diabetes test. Earlier in the week, before my tests, one of the training companies to whom I subcontract had sent me a year's supply of chocolate bars for training course prizes in a suitcase. I'm not saying I ate an entire suitcase of chocolate bars in a week but I taste-tested a fair few. I suspect it may have skewed the results somewhat.

I'm up for re-testing in a few months and it is timely, as I'm reading all this research about sugar and obesity. You can probably ascertain from my photo in this book that I am not obese, far from it. I'm also a gym rat, always have been. And yet a simple, free and routine test gave me a red flag. Accurate or not, this approach is wise. Most days, I consider myself a reasonably smart guy but I wasn't smart enough to proactively seek the test myself. I was lucky.

I was also lucky to grow up in a fairly poor family. The treats and sodas and movie candy that I lavish on my own kids, we never had. Once I got an income of my own, I made very good friends with a range of fastfood outlets and cheap and nasty high-calorie / low-nutritional value foodlike substances. My basic diet was pretty good but it was augmented with a lot of crap. I was (and am) lean but I was *fat on the inside*.

In 1993, an analysis called *The Actual Causes of Death in the United States* was published by epidemiologists William Foege and J. Michael McGinnis. They looked into the factors accounting for the chronic diseases and such that immediately preceded premature deaths. They identified a top ten and it provokes quite a mindset shift. We need to move from thinking about Cancer, Heart Disease, Lung Disease, Stroke and Diabetes as <u>causes</u>. They are <u>effects</u>!

We have substantial influence over everything on their top ten.

Their top three accounts for 66% of the deaths.

38%	Tobacco38%
14%	Diet
14%	Activity patterns
10%	Alcohol
08%	Microbial agents
06%	Toxic agents
4%	Firearms
02%	Sexual behaviour
02%	Motor vehicles
02%	Illicit drug use

David Katz calls this, "Bad use of our feet, forks and fingers... Feet, forks, and fingers are the master levers of medical destiny." If we took wiser control over our feet, forks and fingers, we could eliminate or hugely mitigate 76% of our chances of premature death and end-of-life decline.

If you're the sort of person who is reading this book (and you are) then you'll soon start noticing more media coverage of the debate between the established official wisdom that fat is mostly bad for you and it is supposed to make you fat and sick and is especially guilty when it comes to heart disease. And if you eat nothing but kilograms of butter a day then this will probably be true for you. But no one does that and we cannot look at one factor in isolation.

Most of those diseases of affluence killing us and rendering our last years unhealthy and miserable are accelerated by internal inflammation and insulin-resistance. It's worth investing a bit of time here with a primer on insulin without getting too technical.

Dr Grant Schofield from AUT University sums it up, "Insulin is a hormone produced by the pancreas which helps move glucose into cells. It is essential for life. Sometimes cells become resistant to insulin so it is harder to move the glucose onto those cells. This is called insulin resistance. Insulin resistance is a normal and useful human condition, at least in our natural (ancestral) environment."

When our caveman ancestors were hungry, their bodies prioritised the brain and any spare glucose floating around got directed to our brain. The brain doesn't need insulin to absorb the glucose for energy whereas most of our other cells do. So, with no glucose for fuel, those other cells burn fat. In anticipation of these hungry times, those caveman bodies stored fat. This was a great system for survival when times were unpredictable and we didn't know for sure where or when our next meal was coming from. Or if we were going to be something else's next meal!

There were good reasons to have that spare fuel go to the brain:

- Grunt, need to think how to get food or I'll die,

- Grunt, need to think how to avoid getting eaten by something else,

- Grunt, my species really needs me to breed but now is not a good time for kids because of the drought and the famine, so best I focus on the food and survival thing right now and maybe worry about getting jiggy later. Oh... and grunt.

Problem! We're no longer cavemen. If you can buy this book (and you should) then you can buy food. Droughts might affect the price of your meals but you're getting fed. So, that insulin resistance which has been such a good friend to us for millennia is now a problem. It can get activated by modern influences, not just old-fashioned seasonal food scarcity. Most everything you are surrounded by turns on insulin resistance. Grant Schofield rattled off a list, "Stress, poor sleep, too much exercise, too little exercise, high sugar diet, high Omega 6/trans fat diet, poor gut micro biome, high alcohol diet, obesity, smoking, pollution, other environmental toxins, too much sun, too little sun..."

This is where the debate begins around fats versus carbs. I recommend you read up on it, starting with http://profgrant.com/and skipping to http://www.heartfoundation.org.nz/healthy-living/healthy-eating.

Everyone you know will chip in their opinion and confuse you even more, probably resulting with continued behavioural inertia. I'll expand in the 'Eat' section but my advice would be to disregard every diet that has a book someone is trying to sell you and every diet with a label. Just eat food and stop eating non-food. Food exists. The most you need to do to it is cook it. Meat is food. A carrot is food. Non-food needs to be manufactured. Cake is non-food, even a cake you make yourself. Same goes for pasta.

Dr John Tickell, after laughing off the relevance of worrying about the G.I. levels of food, writes of his own measure: H.I. (Human interference.) I'd have to agree that the greater the human interference in anything between its natural existence and your mouth, the less of a food it actually is and the better off you'd be without it.

There's quite an illuminating infographic doing the rounds of the internet with pictures of all-natural foods like eggs, bananas and blueberries with a list of ingredients as if each was a manufactured item. No surprise that the miraculous blueberry contains 10% sugars (fructose, glucose and sucrose.) There's also methionine and butryraldehyde. I have no idea what they are and neither do you without a quick Google and you're not doing that regularly in the aisles of the fruit shop or supermarket. One is an amino acid and the other is a naturally-occurring flavour. I'm guessing those are good things. I like blueberries.

People like and for any kind of liveable life, people probably need *simplifications*. Obviously my avoidance of non-food guideline and Tickell's H.I. guideline are massive oversimplifications. Wine for example is manufactured, even if you make it yourself, and there's evidence that a couple of glasses a day does you good physically, mentally and socially. But, as a general rule, for the most part, you'd be best to aim for at least half your food being plants, coming as close to natural as possible.

Now you and I both know that you and I are still going to eat cake and pasta. We're grown-ups with free will and disposable income and we can and we will. I'm choosing to eat less of it and less frequently. Nevermind how it affects you in the long-run, how productive, alert and energetic do you feel after cake or pasta? What proportion of your diet is cake, pasta, soda, pizza, breads, etc? Your choices are yours. How are they working out for you so far? How'd they work out for your Dad?

This book has given me, and now you, a huge range of tools and motivators to get myself on a better track physically so I can live longer, better and more productively for my family and myself. There is no one silver bullet. It'd be great if three blueberries a day could solve all our problems. There is a wide range of things you can do, do better, do more or stop doing to set yourself up better for your own reasons - even something as simple and mundane as flossing your teeth.

As I'll stress now and later, I'm not advocating any one particular exclusive diet / ideology / philosophy but I am cherry-picking ideas from lots of them. (Or blueberry-picking?) I'm certainly not suggesting we live like cavemen but genetically and physically, we are not far removed from them, so maybe we can re-adopt selected practices that are in synch with our natural body's design and systems? Mark Sisson's book 'The Primal Blueprint lays out 10 rules which are pretty sensible:

1. Eat Plants and Animals

2. Avoid Poisonous Things

3. Move Frequently at a Slow Pace

4. Lift Heavy Things

5. Sprint Once in a While

6. Get Adequate Sleep

7. Play

8. Get Adequate Sunlight

9. Avoid Stupid Mistakes

10. Use Your Brain

Point 9 is a good one that I don't expand on much but needs to be mentioned. It doesn't matter how fit you are if you get hit by a bus crossing the street without looking. Any damage you do to yourself has the capacity to keep on damaging you for the rest of your life. Injuries, illnesses, infections all create unnecessary inflammation and tax your systems, even the little ones. Sure, you need to build up resistances and immunities but that is going to happen anyway without you going out of your way with carelessness and self-neglect.

There is a correlation, not necessarily causative, between gum disease and memory loss. It's a pretty good idea to practise effective dental hygiene for its own sake but with this suggestion comes a greater motivation. Maybe the same germs in your head attacking your gums beat up your brain too? Maybe people who don't have their act together to look after their teeth also display other behaviours that hurt themselves physically and mentally. A 2007 study published in the Journal of Periodontology found that severe gum disease leads to higher levels of the inflammatory marker C-reactive protein.

Founding director of the New England Centenarian Study Dr Tom Perls said, "The older you get, the healthier you've been." Whatever so-called longevity genes we've got operating (or not operating) inside us, they provide for a vigorous life throughout, not just extra years tagged on at the end. And, ideally, you'd like to avoid ailments throughout your life. Although there are falling rates of hospitals actually conducting post mortems, with only 10% of hospital deaths having them done in the US, they do reveal that 40% of clinical diagnoses were inaccurate. Ouch!

You can take Perls' online calculator at www.livingto100.com. My results claim that I might clock in at 98. I need to eat less red meat, eat less sugar, floss more and get a couple more super-close friends.

A Harvard longitudinal study of 2357 men with an average age of 72 looked for lifestyle choices that would increase their odds of making it to 90. They found that once you got to 70, being a non-smoking regular exerciser with no hypertension, diabetes or obesity, you had a 54% chance of making it to 90.

The 2009 European Prospective Investigation into cancer and Nutrition (EPIC) studied 25,153 people, focusing on their health and behaviours, especially:

- Smoking,
- Weight,
- Physical activity,
- Diet.

At the risk of stating and repeating the bloody obvious, here's the magic formula for health and longevity from a physical point of view:

[Never smoke] + [Keep your body mass index under 30] + [Take part if at least 3.5 hours a week of physical activity] + [Maintain a diet where 50% is fruit, vegetables and wholegrains] = **80% reduction in the risk of any chronic disease ever**

Contrast the above with the U.S. Centre for Disease Control projecting that by 2050, one in three American adults will have diabetes. And of course, diabetes, as bad as it is in its own right, is also a gateway disease. It's not the zombie apocalypse they need to worry about.

Here's the quick précis on BMI. The BMI or Body Mass Index was devised in Belgium in 1830 so it might be due an update. There are a few anomalies which people often cite to discredit the BMI. High performance athletes can often turn out to be technically obese. But for most people, it's a pretty good guide. It takes height <u>and</u> weight into account.

BMI = Weight in kilograms / Height in metres squared

For example, when I started writing this book I was 92 kilograms, so my BMI was: 27.2 = 92kg / (1.84m x 1.84m)

After a few weeks of writing this book, my weight is now 81kg, so now my BMI is: 23.9 = 81kg / 1.84m x 1.84m)

These next few paragraphs might seem out of place in the 'Physical' section but the brain-body connection is so entwined, it may as well go here, especially when exercising, eating properly and getting into good sleep habits are more about the

51

mental process of changing our own behaviours than about the purely physical.

Chip & Dan Heath in their book 'Switch: How To Change Things When Change Is Hard' use a powerful metaphor to describe the relationship between our rational and emotional minds. Our emotional mind is the elephant and our rational mind is that elephant's rider. That elephant is big and powerful and can do whatever it wants whenever it wants and, sure, the rider will eventually get the elephant under control but in the meantime, a lot of damage can be done.

Psychologist Roy Baumeister is an expert on willpower. He showed that willpower is a finite and exhaustible resource. In one experiment, groups of people were given some brainteasers to do that increased in difficulty. But, before they got to do the tests, they were put through some form filling in a waiting area. Available in the waiting area as snacks were carrot sticks and candy. Half the people were allowed the candy and half the carrots. Those who had to consume their willpower not eating the candy ended up giving up sooner in the brainteasers. They had used up all their willpower. Ironically, other than time, the only 'fuel' Baumeister has been able to show bolsters our willpower reserves... is sugar.

Other experiments in this area have suggested that our self discipline is less like a fuel and more like a muscle and if we exercise it then it can become stronger. Later in this book, I'll show you BJ Fogg's work on behaviour change via what he calls 'Tiny habits.' That approach takes time and, meanwhile, we have to deal with a rampaging elephant.

Individually and collectively as a society, our eating has changed in recent decades and the drivers are largely economic. So too is the impact:

	% Income Spent On Food	*% Income Spent On Health*
1960	17.5%	05.2%
2008	09.9%	16.0%

Self supervision is exhausting, literally, so buddy systems will prove useful to keep you on track and to keep you honest. If you're trying to achieve a goal or behaviour change in whatever area, having a friend with a shared commitment is a powerful lever. We'll learn more about this tool later as well.

Let's move onto the first of the 12 controls and the first of the three Physical ones - Moving.

5.3.1.1

Move

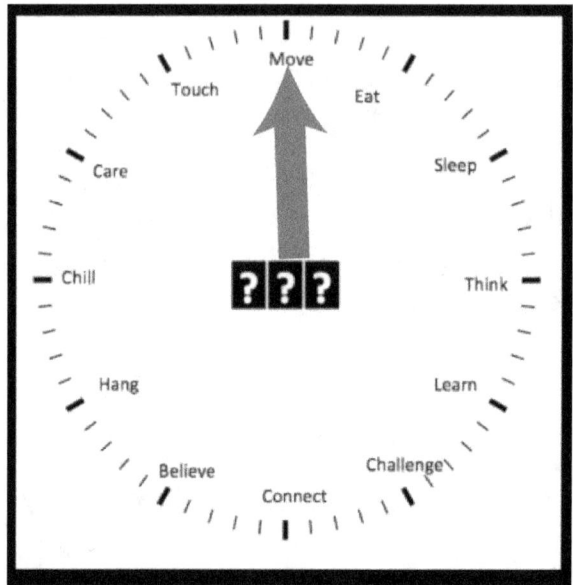

Sitting is as bad as smoking,

Poor movement can be a sign of potential health issues,

Exercise is not as important as having activity as part of your everyday life.

"I believe that the good lord gave us a finite number of heartbeats and I'm damned if I'm going to use mine running up and

A clinical review from doctors at the University of Alabama at Birmingham suggests that mobility limitations are a litmus test for healthy aging and urges primary care physicians to take a more aggressive role in ascertaining the mobility of their patients. They suggest that doctors should ask all patients two questions: for health or physical reasons, do you have difficulty climbing up 10 steps or walking 400m at a brisk pace; and because of underlying health or physical reasons, have you modified the way you climb 10 steps or walk 400m?

Can you sit on the floor, then get up again without using your hands, knees or elbows? Go on, try it right now. The physical inability to do that, or struggle to barely do that, has been cited as an indicator of potential heart problems. Such is the inter-connectedness of our physical systems. Muscular strength, balance, bone density – none of these things are our hearts, but they can help or hurt our heart, depending on how we maintain them and they give us constant information on how things are going inside.

Dr Steven Blair in studies with both the Cooper Clinic in Dallas and the University of South Carolina tracked thousands of people over dozens of years. They determined that fitness levels (not fatness levels) are significant predictors of mortality. Poor fitness accounts for sixteen percent of all deaths. Move it or lose it. It's never too late to start to reap benefits but it's always too soon to stop. Some people say that they're too old to exercise but the truth is that they're too old not to exercise.

A University of Hong Kong study made similar findings. Twenty percent of deaths in people over 35 could be attributed to physical inactivity, greater than the risk caused by smoking. (Of course, that doesn't bode well for smokers who are also physically inactive.) Physical inactivity increases risks for the following causes of death:

Cause	*Men*	*Women*
Cancer	Up 45%	Up 28%
Respiratory Illness	Up 92%	Up 75%
Heart disease	Up 52%	Up 28%

Modern medicine is amazing but can it be improved on, or even replaced, in some instances?

A study published in the British Medical Journal by scientists from the London School of Economics, Harvard Medical School, Harvard Pilgrim Health Care Institute and Stanford University reviewed the results of 305 previous trials with over three hundred thousand people to see if physical activity was as effective as drugs at preventing death among people with coronary heart disease, rehabilitation from stroke, treatment for heart failure and prevention of diabetes. "There was no difference between exercise and drug interventions for the people with coronary heart disease and for the prevention of diabetes." You don't hear about this because pharmaceutical companies can't sell you a bottle of walking. Although, one of the authors Huseyin Naci was at pains to stress, "The results of our study by no means imply that people should stop taking their medications, especially without consulting their doctors."

The BBC reported a study in the British Journal of Sports Medicine that followed 3,500 healthy people at or around retirement age. Those who took up exercise were three times more likely to remain healthy over the next eight years than their sedentary peers. Exercise cut the risk of heart disease, stroke, diabetes, Alzheimer's disease and depression.

The University of Bath studied a group of 26 healthy young men. All exercised regularly. None were obese. Baseline health assessments, including biopsies of fat tissue, confirmed that each had normal metabolisms and blood sugar control, with no symptoms of incipient diabetes. The scientists then asked all their volunteers to impair their great health by doing a lot of sitting and eating way too much. But half the volunteers had to do a hard-out 45 minute treadmill session a day. Other than that session, they lay around all the rest of the day.

The New York Times reported the results: After only a week, the young men who had not exercised displayed a significant and unhealthy decline in their blood sugar control, and, equally worrying, their biopsied fat cells seemed to have developed a malicious streak. Those cells, examined using sophisticated genetic testing techniques, were now overexpressing various genes that may contribute to unhealthy metabolic changes and underexpressing other genes potentially important for a well-functioning metabolism.

But the volunteers who had exercised once a day, despite comparable energy surpluses, were not similarly afflicted. Their blood sugar control remained robust, and their fat cells exhibited far fewer of the potentially undesirable alterations in gene expression than among the sedentary men.

"Exercise seemed to completely cancel out many of the changes induced by overfeeding and reduced activity," said Dylan Thompson, a professor of health sciences at the University of Bath and senior author of the study.

Fitness for health isn't about gyms and jogging as much as it is about a physically active lifestyle that exerts strong system-wide effects on our body. Rather than exercising for the sake of it, make changes to your lifestyle and environment that encourages you to move. Ride a bicycle. Walk. Park your car further away. Use the stairs. Chances are, you'll sustain that physical activity longer than most people sustain their gym membership.

The 'runner's high' that we experience when we do break through the initial tough bit of exercise is due to brain chemicals called endocannabinoids. (Yes, it's one of *those* cannabinoids...) Some suppose this was an evolutionary outcome to support us back in the day when if we wanted dinner, we had to chase it and catch it. And it might be why stoners get the munchies.

People in western economies sit 9.3 hours a day and that doesn't include sleeping.

Physical inactivity leads to muscle and bone weakness, immune system compromises, narrowing of arteries, metabolic decline, central nervous system compromise and general frailty. Sitting can be as bad as smoking. They should print warnings on couches and office chairs. Even if the chair is perfectly primed by a professional Ergonomist and made safe from any posture or health and safety issue, the very act of being sedentary and sitting for long periods is not what humans are suited for. In fact, it's the opposite.

Between 1945 and 1995, the average adult daily calorie expenditure fell 800 calories. So the amount of moving we do each day has reduced by 800 calories, thanks to cars and machines and washing machines and so forth. 800 calories is the equivalent of **a ten mile walk**! In 1960, 50% of jobs required at least moderate physical activity. Today it is only 20%. Two thirds of desk workers eat lunch at their desk.

The Mayo Clinic takes credit for labelling a phenomenon it calls 'Non-Exercise Activity Thermogenesis' (NEAT.) I call it moving. Doing stuff burns calories. You don't have to join a gym, swim an ocean or run marathons religiously. Make a bed, walk the stairs and stand while talking on the phone. They're also licensing devices to be NEAT-certified to measure and motivate people, including special underwear. I presume the underwear is more about the measuring than the motivation?

We need to develop lifelong patterns of enjoyable activity.

Avoid, prevent or lessen fall risks with balance exercises. These don't have to be yoga or tai-chi, though you'd probably benefit from doing that with a group socially. You can do them at home while watching TV to lessen the negative effects of being a couch potato.

Here's a few:

- Walk an imaginary line on the floor heel-to-toe while not looking at your feet, just like a cop suspecting you of drink-driving in a movie in the 1970s,

- Stand in that karate kid stance when he had the broken leg (but you don't have to leap and kick a blond guy in the head),

- Get off and on the couch using only one leg. Change legs. Repeat. (Don't go and get Dorritos between times – not even the new buffalo wings flavour when you got that 3-for-$5 deal at the supermarket.)

According to Oscar Franco of Erasmus MC University, walking thirty minutes a day for five days a week can add eighteen months to your life.

Sex is like cellphone credit – use it or lose it. Some research reckons sex three times a week can add two years to your life, bolstering natural levels of DHEA, HGH, immunoglobin-A and Oxytocin. Oxytocin is not only a painkiller but has some psychological benefits I'll expand on later in the 'Love' section. "Men who ejaculate at least seven times a week in their 20s were found to be over a third less likely to develop aggressive prostate cancer in later life than men who only muster three," says study author Professor Graham Giles from the Cancer Council Victoria. It is best if it is real sex with a real person though. Orgasms are healthy however you come by them but one-on-one consensual sex maximising skin-on-skin contact yields four hundred times the positive hormones etc. To try and achieve that by yourself, well, who has the time?

One book described orgasms using computer lingo, as a means of "rebooting your brain." Well, every time you ring a help desk, the first question is always, "Is it turned on?"

Couples who have sex at least four times a week look more than 10 years younger than the average adult, concluded a Royal Edinburgh Hospital study. "Pleasure derived from sex is a crucial factor in preserving youth due to the release of adrenaline, dopamine, and norepinephrine," says Neuropsychologist Dr David Weeks, who conducted the study. "Plus, sex triggers human growth hormone which combats free radicals from pollution, and exposure to other damaging environmental factors. This helps preserve skin cell walls and relax muscles which could otherwise cause wrinkles."

A study in the journal *Biological Psychology* found men who had had sex the previous night responded better to stressful situations. All down to the soothing effect of another person's touch, says Professor Stuart Brody, sexual psychologist from the University of Paisley. "A great deal of research has shown touch has a naturally calming effect," says Brody. "And being touched by someone you care about significantly increases that effect." Apart from the pleasurable sensation, researchers found touch actually reduces levels of the stress hormone cortisol.

UK Men's Health Magazine will spell out the sexual positions and activities that will optimise norepinephrine production. At least, I think so. My friend told me.

The body's physical and mental systems interact. For example, aerobic exercise stimulates the production of Brain Derived Neurotrophic factor (BDNF) which supports the brain's existing and new synapses and neurons. Columbia University's Medical Centre in New York ran a study that found that the risk of Alzheimers is reduced by a third in the physically active. Add to that physical activity a diet rich in fruit and vegetables, and that risk reduces by a total of 60%.

A study published in 2010 in the American Journal of Epidemiology conducted by the American Cancer Society's observed thousands of people between 1993 and 2006. They concluded, "Sitting for extended periods is a health risk as insidious as smoking or over-exposure to the sun." Melbourne's International Diabetes Institute found that even two hours daily exercise does not make up for the other twenty two hours if they're motionless. "Blood levels of C-reactive protein (a marker of inflammation) were twice as high in people who spent four or more hours a day in front of a screen than people spending two or less."

I interviewed Dr Grant Schofield of AUT University's Human Potential centre. I've included more excerpts of his passionate smarts in the 'Eat' section. In walking into his office in the *Millennium Institute of Sport and Health* on Auckland's North Shore, the first thing that struck me was the view of the athletics tracks outside his office window – a great metaphor for moving if ever there was one. The second thing I noticed was the furniture, as I made the traditional foray to find a seat to continue our chat. I didn't recognise any of it.

My experience with workplace ergonomic furniture came from managing a call centre where the mission was to get people seated as comfortably as possible, whilst minimising the potential for any physical harms that might occur from poor angles and heights and such of the furniture. I never knew then that the very act of prolonged sitting was, itself, harmful.

Grant proudly described his team's self-made furniture as 'UN-ergonomic. The stools, if they could be called that, were boxy and the seat component was angled. It was not only not designed to be sat in for long periods, it was purposefully designed to encourage people to get off it frequently. The height and layout of the 'desks' makes standing very practical and the overall layout provokes efficient movement.

Later on in the 'Work' section, I'll suggest a concept called 'Walking Meetings.' Having a running track outside would be ideal for those. But not everyone has a running track at their work, nor purpose-built UN-ergonomic furniture. If that's you, your need to move is going to have to be self-managed. But if you can re-jig your physical environment, it's proven to be the most effective way to instigate changes and maintain the new wiser behaviours.

If you truly feel that you're absolutely chained to your desk then there's always the option of 'Deskercise.' Here are a few variations, using your chair or desk as tools for movement and that won't get your 'LA Law' fashion work clothes all sweaty:

- Incline push-ups against desk,

- Tricep dips with chair behind you,

- Standing up off your chair using only one leg,

- Alternate knee-rises while seated,

- Plyometrics – push sideways against the interior walls of your desk like you're The Hulk trying to break your legs out of prison.

If you need safety warning about your chair being on wheels and so forth, then I should probably tell you:

- Coffee is hot,

- Don't use that new hairdryer while in the bath

An Australian study of 12,000 people found that, after the age of 25, each hour of TV watching decreased life expectancy by 22 minutes. A cigarette only reduced it by 11 minutes! Best not smoke while watching TV then, that's for sure. Again, it's not TV per se that's the problem, it's the associated social disconnection, mindless eating and sitting motionless. Average six hours of that kind of TV watching a day and it'll take five years off your life. How can you add activity to your TV watching? Suggestions include wobbleboards, exercycles, light dumbbells and resistance bands. Certainly the latter can be stored wherever the remote control lives and be easily accessed for a few plyometrics with the coffee table. Even fidgeting is better than sitting still.

'Breaking Bad' was a classic and well-produced TV show. At fifty or so episodes, was it worth losing 18 hours of my life on top of the time I spent watching it? 'Geordie Shore' is definitely not.

The Baltimore Longitudinal Study on Aging found some good news for couch potatoes who never bother to start any physical efforts because they know they'll never run a marathon. The biggest gains in health from physical activity are not accrued at the top end of the fitness scale. The biggest gains are from the first steps – from being a zero-effort couch potato to being a 10-minute-a-day walker. Oh and get some good shoes – they lessen any risk of inflammation to your joints and back.

You don't need to start triathlons or join a gym, although the social aspects of that and the routine might be helpfully encouraging for some. They are for me. My weekly basketball game is highly social and physically akin to my caveman ancestors' sporadic hunting outbursts.

You do need to crank out thirty to sixty minutes of activity five times a week that combines aerobic work, balance and muscle conditioning. Try deliberately inconveniencing yourself so you have to go downstairs to fetch the laundry basket. If you have to go get a latté, go to the 2nd closest café. Park further away so there is at least a bit of a stroll at the start and end of your work day. Get off your butt every twenty minutes and try to automate that. We're all tethered to smartphones these days so have a regular alarm set to vibrate to remind you to move.

This does make a difference when it all adds up:

	Average daily Steps	*Obesity Rate*
USA	5117	34%
Australia	9695	16%

Studies show that a mere twenty minutes of moderate activity significantly improves your mood in the subsequent twelve hours. Find others to be supportive and move with you.

I'm a latecomer to, but a fan of, the benefits of being a gardener: 45 minutes of gardening will burn the same number of calories as a 30 minute aerobics class,

- Better sleepers,

- Lower risk of osteoporosis,

- Lower risk of diabetes,

Improved coordination, balance and strength means fewer accidents and better recovery from falls in later life,

The fresh food you grow is the best source of nutrients you'll ever get,

It's a project with purpose that multiple generations within a family can share and bond over,

- Save money and spare money is always good for health,

- Reduced anxiety,

- Sense of purpose,

- A routine / ritual and your body and mind like those,

No jogging required.

Gardening and yoga are great. Do yoga in a garden. With others.

> *"Every hour of TV we watch reduces our life expectancy by 22 minutes. One cigarette only reduces it 11. In fairness to TV, it's the sitting that does the harm so be sure to be active TV watchers by miming along with the action on TV. That's what I did with **Breaking Bad**. Unfortunately, I killed my entire family. Lucky I wasn't watching 'Geordie Shore.'" – Terry Williams, 'The Grin Reaper' comedy show*

5.3.1.2

Eat

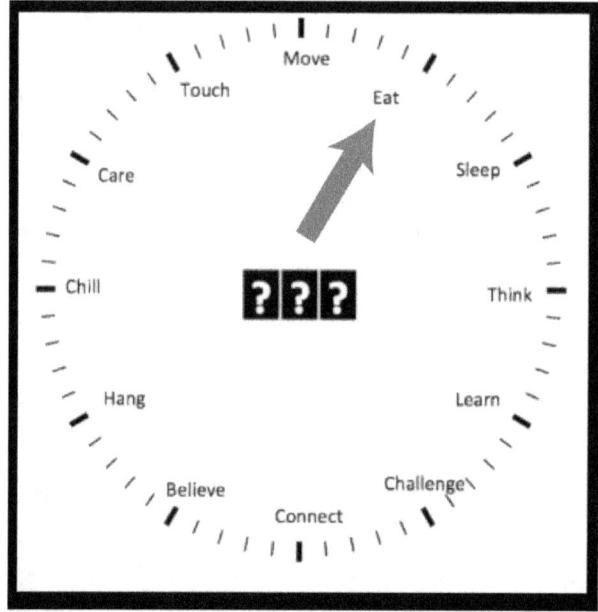

You will never undo through exercise the damage you do by eating poorly. Whatever your current condition, you can eat yourself better,

Your kids see what & how you eat.

New Zealand's All Black rugby team is a pretty successful brand, I would have thought. Research company Colmar-Brunton run an annual survey of which New Zealand brands people are most fond of. The All Blacks – our national sport's national team with a win record perpetually over 80% - were 3rd in 2013. Ahead of them in 2nd place was Tip-Top Ice Cream and in 1st place was Whittakers Chocolate. People in New

Zealand don't wake up in the middle of the night very much anymore to go watch the All Blacks play England but I bet lots of people get up for ice cream and / or chocolate. Also in the top 10 were Cadbury's chocolate and L&P soft drinks. The findings declared, "The best brands evoke positive childhood memories and provide tangible links to those memories - they are known and trusted as well as loved." This is what your brain is up against while it is trying to eat better.

The Millennium Gym and high performance sports centre was a sponsor of my 2013 comedy festival show. In talking with their marketing people, it fell out of the conversation that for many gym members in my age bracket, attending the gym was, "an act of penance." My demographic has to add notches to extend their belts but would like to continue their beer drinking and pie-munching lifestyles. I can eat x if I do y. Exercise is great as we've just covered in the 'Move' section but the main control we have over our life and health spans is the control 'Eat.'

A brisk three mile walk will burn for an average adult 275 calories. Eating one donut will add 360. You will not win the penance race at the gym. To attempt to do will force you into over-exercising and you'll reap the negative consequences like inflammation etc that damage you, age you and open the door for other maladies.

Our ancestors feasted whenever the opportunity presented itself. In Paleolithic times, opportunities were few and far between. These days you turn your head and someone will shove a pie in your mouth, with promises of cronuts for afters. Mmmm cronuts...

It's confusing if you do start to look for information about how to eat better. Vested interests and competing and contradictory viewpoints abound. Plus, sometimes, many of us can be a little lazy or believe what we find convenient to believe. Two hours at the gym will not make up for a day that is otherwise inactive and filled with cronuts.

Even me using the term 'Paleolithic' earlier has the potential to be contentious. There is an industry around the concept of the Paleo diet or primitive or primal. Let's live as cavemen did, they never got fat, say one group. Critics respond, yeah but they all died at 30. Proponents retort, yeah but that was because of massive infant mortality, infections and poor hygiene and such, not their diet. You weren't there so you don't know.

I'm not suggesting we emulate a caveman lifestyle. For a start, dragging women home by their hair is frowned upon these days. But we modern peeps need to do something to deal with how our bodies' systems become dysregulated with today's over-abundance of food and under-commitment to physical activity. This is preventing us from enjoying the extra longevity technology has gifted us. I can't hunt a mammoth and I'd prefer not to kill my steak but I am prepared to eat a wider variety of veges and stand while watching basketball on TV. Of all the themed lifestyles out there, I quite like large chunks of their thinking. It's hard to argue with, "Don't eat crap" and "Get off your butt." Eating wholefoods in as close to their natural state is not just ancient wisdom, its wise wisdom.

But then, some of their thinking suggests pizza lovers can get over their love affair with that refined-carb white-flour base by making 'meatzza' instead. I'll let your imagination work out what 'meatzza' might entail. It's more mainstream than you might think. Google "Meatzza" and the first entry is a Nigella Lawson recipe.

At the other end of the scale (or scales) is the YouTube Sensation 'Epic Meal Time.' www.epicmealtime.com A group of young American men video themselves constructing massive monuments to fat-laden, sugar-soaked self-destruction. They are over-the-top entertainment in a foul and disgusting kind of way but it is an unashamed celebration of everything that is killing Americans and how it is happening. They are gloriously self-aware as they create a giant lasagne made from dozens of burgers bought from McDonalds, Burger King, Wendys and others layered into large catering-sized trays then smothered in extra special sauce, bacon and cheese. The lasagne episode alone has over 21,580,000 views. Three of which were mine. You cannot watch this just once.

Everything gets bacon added. Even sweet things like their giant energy bar. Their sushi filled with cut-up burgers, fries and popcorn chicken replaces the more traditional seaweed sheet with bacon. In fairness, they do have a calorie meter running in realtime on screen as they add layer after layer off ill-advised ingredients. These heroes of gluttony have a catchphrase, "We make your dreams come true and then we eat them."

We don't have to eat like it's the Paleolithic era but we'd be better off eating like it was 1959.

People believe what they want to believe and see the evidence they choose to see that supports their beliefs. This is well supported Psychology 101. That's why I have 12 controls and they're in a particular order but it's not a chronological order or in order of importance. I think for you to succeed in the long-run in achieving your extra 10 productive years, you're going to have to have the support and the motivation from those you love and are connected with. The foundation of all this effort are your **social** controls. Then you need to get your own individual head right with your **mental** controls. Only then will you be able to make those **physical** controls stick and become effective over time. I'm certain so many efforts at diets and other self improvements fall down because there isn't that solid foundation.

One of the drivers behind such folk as the Primal Blueprint people is their tremendous sense of community. I like some of what they're saying but I'm not especially promoting them however they have a powerfully supportive network, highly enabled by the internet. Yes, there is a company with a personality selling things behind it but their social support set-up is a great idea executed well. Whatever you set your mind towards achieving after reading this book, your odds of success will greatly swell if you muck in with others.

Beliefs are sometimes surprisingly disappointing. Surveys show that 25% of people believe 'Fair Trade' food products contain fewer calories. Fair Trade deserves a halo but not inherently a health halo. 'Organic' is not necessarily healthy either. They can make organic high fructose corn syrup. But people are willing to pay 23% more for a label that says 'Organic.' Again, organic is a good thing and deserves a premium but that has nothing to do with health. Yet, we transfer ticks in our minds to everything about a product and the marketing departments know this. The boxes that you most need to read the nutritional info on are the boxes that scream out the loudest a single health claim. Nothing says we've got too much sugar and artificial colours than a cartoon character yelling about a teaspoon of added fibre.

Dwight Howard is an NBA all-star basketball centre. Almost seven feet tall and a chiselled athlete, he once won the All Star dunk contest on a custom built hoop he bought in with a height of twelve feet off the ground instead of the standard ten feet. He is the last guy you'd expect to have health problems from what he eats and, at age 27, we'd all expect to be able to chow down on whatever whenever and burn it off, especially when you're a high-performance athlete. His nickname is Superman.

After two seasons of injuries and back surgery, his recovery was slow and disappointing for himself and his team at the time, the Los Angeles Lakers. As part of the battery of medical tests he went through, and money was no object, they tested his blood. The Daily Mail reported that Dr Cate Shanahan, a nutrition specialist recalled seeing the telltale signs of sugar addiction, "Spikes in energy followed by crashes and erratic motor skills that were indicative of nerves misfiring."

Howard was famous for being a poor free-throw shooter. Opposing teams would often implement a strategy called 'Hack-A-Howard' where they would intentionally foul him at the end of close games as the odds of him making free throws was less than the threat he posed in general play. One of the other symptoms of his sugar-fuelled malaise was swollen hands and that will negatively impact your free throws. Just from candy and soda, Howard consumed the equivalent of 24 Hershey bars a day. And if he couldn't burn it off, then you and I certainly can't.

Following his new sugar-sensible eating lifestyle, his blood sugar levels dropped 80% within weeks and his body fat halved. There's no radical fad diet. He stopped eating non-food and started eating only actual food. He says that his new teammates think he's crazy for opting for beetroot over burgers, but he concluded: "I just made a commitment. You've got to start doing little things now that will prolong your career. I can tell once I've had something bad, my body feels different." Substitute the word "career" with "life" and I reckon Dwight just summed up the purpose of this book.

I'm not a fan of whatever superfood dejour is doing the rounds of the media. Blueberries are great but, by themselves, they're not going to save your life, do your taxes and ward off vampires. Neither are micro-greens or whatever someone comes up with next who also happens to be selling them. Don't obsess about finding and eating superfoods. How about just eating food? And not eating things that aren't food? You don't need a scientist, a Doctor or a 70s sitcom actress to tell you not to eat partially hydrogenated vegetable oil or high fructose corn syrup. Yet many of us eat it and are unaware of how much nor of the accumulated consequences.

It's amazing how we're programmed. Without thinking, I capitalised the word "Doctor" in the previous paragraph but not scientist or sitcom actress.

If you read as many books on health and aging as I have in researching this book, you'd get sick – sick of miracle cures being dangled and marketed. If we all just inhaled, bathed in, or injected a blend of mitochondria, CoQ10, resveratrol, bioidentical hormones, alpha-lipoic acid and Vitamin E, we'd be set for life as youthful superstars. It's actually simpler, cheaper and a lot more scientifically-based to shut up and eat your fruit and vegetables. Trust me. I'm not trying to sell you fruit and vegetables and this book isn't published by a company under the control of the multinational broccoli corporations.

In his book 'The Wellness revolution', Paul Pilzer outlines the extensive business opportunities and entrepreneurial profits to be made with the billions of dollars consumers are going to throw at staying young and trying not to die - selling water, augmenting waters, growing soy, so many meds and new types of insurance. But wait! There's more!

And he's right. And in the minds of many businesses, you are nothing but a wallet on legs and any new drive on your part towards wellness is just another way for them to transfer some wealth from you to them. Every time you hear a news item about health, apply a cynical ear and ask, "Who stands to profit from this?"

An older friend of mine posted on FaceBook a blog post about coconut oil and how one woman's aged mother was brought back from the brink of dementia by its miraculous restorative properties. The internet and crowd-sourcing of science may one day lead to surges forward in development but meanwhile it's a great place for lies, manipulation, misinformation and cognitive dissonance. What there is evidence of is that (if you subscribe to the prevailing but increasingly challenged official wisdom that fats are bad for you) it's the plant with the highest levels of unhealthy saturated fats. If you want unhealthier fat, you have to go catch yourself a pig. It may be that the blog author's mum did take coconut oil and did recover. That is not cause and effect. However, the extensive links to coconutoil.com on the blog would lead me to suspect that the blog's author might not be super independent.

In what's believed to be the first clinical trial of its kind, the University of South Florida Health Byrd Alzheimer's Institute enrolled 65 individuals with mild to moderate Alzheimer's to measure the effects of coconut oil - versus placebo - on the disease. There is currently no clinical data showing the benefits of coconut oil on the prevention and treatment of dementia, Lead researcher Mary Newport - whose husband Steve was diagnosed with Alzheimer's at age 51 - said she began to see improvements after starting him on four teaspoons of coconut oil per day. Canada's CTV News reported Newport as saying, "Our brains rely on glucose from carbohydrates. But if that isn't available, because we haven't eaten anything or are on a low-carbohydrate diet, then our brain cells switch to using the energy from our fat. This energy comes in the form of small molecules called ketones."

I wonder about research where there is such a conflict of interest in the lead researcher. She hopes for results within a year. I'll have confidence in the results if they can be replicated. That's science not hope and desperation.

That said, getting good fats into you is good for your brain and may well reduce your chances of dementia. I just started using coconut oil sparingly as it smells delightful but my mainstay is extra virgin olive oil.

The whole 'good fats' area is one fraught currently with controversy, confusion and contradictions. It's easy for me to preach "get the good fats into ya" but, if that's all a reader chooses to hear, it'll be a slow, limping and puffed race to a heart attack. Which of the following fats or fat sources do you think are "good"?:

- Almonds,
- Bacon,
- Avocados,
- Salmon,
- Olives,

- Meat,

- Macadamia nuts,

- Eggs,

- Cheese,

- Chocolate

- Butter,

- Cream,

- Olive oil,

- Canola oil,

- Coconut oil

You're not going to like the answer because it's not a simple one. Some fats are less bad than others and some fats are good but only if you maintain a certain ratio of carbohydrates consumption in relation to the fats you consume. Most writings then proceed to start using actual measurement in grams of how much carbohydrate and from sources zzzzzzzzzzz. No one wants to hear that. Who has the time or inclination? I'm writing a book on the subject and I'm a pretty interested and motivated guy but the moment I read of having to measure my dialy carb intake in grams I zzzzzzzz... That's why people look for the quick, simple and easy. The world is full of cautionary tales from people hungry for the simple answer dangled by diet pedlars.

That said, let's give a quick low-down on fat. Fat *per se* doesn't directly make you fat or give you heart attacks. It might if that was all you ate and you did nothing else. Good fats are unrefined animal fats, fat from fish, and select fats from plants, such as avocado, olive, nuts, and tropical oils. They tend to include a higher proportion of saturated or monounsaturated fats or be higher in omega-3s.

Bad fats are vegetable fats such as soy, peanut, corn, safflower, sunflower, and canola oil *that have been refined.* Higher in omega-6 fats, they're very prone to oxidation during processing, which makes them reactive and damaging to your body's systems.

Overall, you'll accrue more benefits from consuming good fats when you limit your processed carbohydrate intake. So, have eggs on toast but without the toast.

Resveratrol is another cautionary tale. Be wary of the media, supposed miracle cures and the profit motive. Resveratrol is a natural phenol that occurs naturally in some plants, such as Japanese Knotweed and, more fortuitously, red wine grapes. In the mid 90s, it was touted as perhaps the reason for the French having better health than the Americans, despite having much the same fat-laden diets. The only tests showing any kind of positive effects were done in test tubes, not on people or even mammals. That didn't stop the scientist behind the research selling his company to *Glaxo Smith Klein* for $US720,000,000.

By the way, the Telomeres people scoff at the Resveratrol people.

> *"There's a name for alternative medicines that work," says Joe Schwarcz, professor of chemistry and the director of the Office for Science and Society at McGill University in Montreal. "It's called medicine."*

If ever you're touted such miracles, check out www.quackwatch.org or www.snopes.com

> *"Alternative medicine is defined as that set of practices that cannot be tested, refuse to be tested, or consistently fail tests." –*
> *Richard Dawkins*

Last year, the fastest growing item on breakfast menus in terms of popularity was... soda...

The Mediterranean Diet is often cited as a good thing and it's hard to argue. There's no soda for breakfast and it's as much about the lifestyle surrounding the diet as it is the diet itself. The word "diet" should probably be left out due to its negative baggage as a label.

I wrote about diets in my first book 'The Guide: How to kiss, get a job & other stuff you need to know'. It's still valid:

I cannot stress highly enough that the only reason diet is a topic in this book is to empower you to be more in control of your quality and quantity of life. By 'diet', I mean "stuff you eat so you live longer and enjoy a better lifestyle"; I don't mean "a prescribed constraint of consumption serving only to lose body mass and enrich whichever charlatan sold you their programme." If any of your friends attempt to give you a diet book, take it. Take that diet book and beat them violently and relentlessly with it. This counts as exercise <u>and</u> stress release at the same time. (That's what friends are for.) The only way to lose fat is to burn more calories as energy than you consume. Anything else is a short-term gimmick leading to a 'diet cycle' with all that weight coming back with a vengeance.

That said, if you've got a gut or your belt notches are giving you negative feedback, it's not just an image problem. The illusion of the 'fit fat' is just that – an illusion. There's nothing wrong with not conforming to some abstract idealised external model of supposed perfection. No one does and it's another way of selling you clothes, foods, programmes and unhappiness. But gut flab is a real problem, not an image problem.

Greg Critser, author of 'Fat Land', specifies the issues: "Excess abdominal fat cells are troublesome in and of themselves. They are, metabolically, the laboratory of the so-called Syndrome X. The Syndrome, first identified by Stanford Endocrinologist Gerald Reaven, acts as the precursor to both Type-2 and, eventually, full-blown insulin-dependent Diabetes. Excess weight is implicated in its progression. This is because insulin-resistant fat cells in the gut produce excess fatty acids, which wreak havoc by attacking the body's vital sugar-processing and fat-processing functions." Hyper-Insulinemia leads to Diabetes. Excess blood fats leads to clogged arteries. Constricted blood flow leads to Hypertension. Just being heavier than your body's structure is used to leads to pressure on the spine, joints and bones and they wear out quicker.

Ironically, eating fat satiates your appetite quicker and, feeling fuller, many consume less overall. Healthy fats help you lose fat by improving metabolism, balancing hormones, and eliminating constant cravings. Healthy fat intake leads to greater gains from strength training. Dry skin and eyes is often caused by a deficiency in fatty acids. Good fat intake allows for higher androgens, better reproductive health and a more active libido. A deficiency of cholesterol and fat in the brain, causes lower levels of the neurotransmitter serotonin contributing to depression. Eating fats in as whole a form as possible (eg nuts) gives you more vitamin D and K2 which promote bone density. Limiting omega-6 oil intake for whole food fats such as olives, avocados, and unprocessed animal fats appears to reduce cancer risk. Fats are not the problem - reduce your heart disease risk and lower your triglycerides by restricting sugar and limiting your carbohydrate intake.

Those Mediterraneans know about good fats. In the deliberate absence of the word "diet", here are some meal aspects of Mediterranean *lifestyles*:

- Meals made from scratch using in-season produce,
- Use of mono-unsaturated olive oil,

- Emphasis on cereals, beans, fresh fruit, variety of vegetables,

- Plenty of herbs and spices,

- Red meat used sparingly and in conjunction with plenty of vegetables,

- Regular fresh fish,

- Occasional treats,

- Red wine,

- Unhurried meals,

- Mealtime shared with family of multiple generations.

Okinawa is another place where diet is cited as a positive influence on health and longevity. Their approach is similar to that above with the addition of green tea, seaweed and soy-based items like miso and tofu.

The Lyon Heart Study in France looked at people having had their first heart attack and the impact of subsequent dietary changes. Those who followed the Mediterranean diet for at least four years, had a 50-70% lower chance of a second heart attack. They had reduced cholesterol, reduced inflammation, reduced levels of type 2 diabetes (which triples your chance of a heart attack) and lower cancer rates.

Stay hydrated. Sometimes we interpret thirst signals from our bodies as hunger. Drink water before you're thirsty. Don't fret about whatever claims there about how much water you should drink – just don't get thirsty. Our bodies are hydro-powered. When I was starting out as a trainer, I went on a course. The trainer got the group into a circle and instructed us to hold hands. At one point he broke the circle and produced a spherical object with a couple of metal contact points. The two people where the circle was broken each touched one of the metal contact points. The object started flashing and buzzing –

powered by the electricity that flows through our bodies and was flowing through the circuit we had formed as a group.

We were then instructed not to drink and we reformed the circle at half hourly intervals. By the ninety minute mark of not drinking, the object barely flashed and buzzed. Such was the impact on the electrical energy of dehydration. And we need that power for our hearts and brains. It's fuelled by water. Drinking sodas or the evil energy drinks won't help and will hurt. Quite apart from their insane sugar levels, they're diuretic and will hasten dehydration. Check out the impact on people. Watch your colleagues who amp up on Red Bull after the initial rush.

My local supermarket now sells water bottles with built-in technology and a screen that provides feedback on how much you've drunk, how much you need to drink and several other variables. Not so much 'feedback' as 'nagging' perhaps? And who says how much you should be drinking? Drink unadulterated water as often as you need to so you never get thirsty. Did you really need me or a talking water bottle to tell you that?

Herbs may have some health benefits. Rosemary and basil are supposed to have anti-inflammatory qualities. Cumin and sage are claimed to mitigate dementia. Cayenne and cinnamon may well limit obesity. Coriander and cinnamon may be sugar regulating. And you know what, even if that isn't true, they taste great and don't do you any harm. Plus, if you are going to the trouble and taking the time to prepare a meal with fresh herbs, it's probably going to be a better meal for you.

Anti-inflammatory foods include fresh wild salmon, walnuts, garlic, onions, blueberries, sweet potatoes, spinach, pineapple, ginger, thumeric, cumin, extra virgin olive oil and pomegranate. Many recommend a baby aspirin daily and there are products now that deliver this in a form less likely to provoke the stomach issues that people with such sensitivities encounter with aspirin. Statin drugs that are often prescribed to patients at risk of inflammation-related heart issues will experience reduced inflammation but such drugs can be immunity suppressants. Pharmacies are _retailers_ – remember that. The U.S. and New Zealand are the only countries in the world that allow direct-to-consumer advertising by drug companies. Whatever happened to Xenical? That was plugged in major advertising campaigns as kind of a morning-after pill for gluttons.

Unless you have a specific and diagnosed deficiency, vitamin supplements will have no proven benefits, be transformed into expensive urine and it is possible that over-consumption causes harm. You'd be better taking that money and spending it on quality fruit and vegetables. (Or buying more of my books.)

I was about to insert a quote at this point about supplements not being the basis of good health and that the most important factors were actually diet and exercise. But then I ran a check on the author of the quote via some of the sceptic and quackwatch sites. The diet and exercise opinion seems valid to me but this is from a guy who makes unsubstantiated claims about vaccines, dentists and cooking pots. The downside of the internet is that anybody's opinion can get greater traction than its merit deserves. Whichever expert your buddy on FaceBook 'likes', check them out via snopes.com or other similar sites to get more of a critical and independent assessment.

It's no good eating great quality and nutritious food if those nutrients don't make it efficiently into your systems via effective digestion. Here is a collection of tips:

- Chew! (Obvious but observe the low chewing habits of people eating in public, especially those soft-food takeaways.)
- Drink water,
- Eat fibre,
- Don't eat before sleeping,

- Eat probiotic yoghurt containing gut-friendly bacteria,

- Slow down, sit down,

- Exercise (Not while you're eating but earlier in the day),

- No more than 2 alcoholic drinks,

- Be self aware – what are your trigger foods?

Calorie restriction switches on Sirtuin1 – the protein encoded by our survival gene SIRT1. Your body tricks itself into thinking it is in the middle of a famine and needs to get into survival mode. So it stores rather than burns fat. This you do not want. So, starving yourself is counter-productive, nevermind the other harms it inflicts on your systems.

According to Dr Pramil Singh of the Loma Linda University School of Public Health, eating meat no more than once a week can add 3 years and 219 days to your life. Doctor Maoshing Ni suggests being a weekday vegetarian and a weekend carnivore, eating like a king by day and a pauper by night, to stop eating dead food and to stop killing our food. The latter relates to cooking techniques. I used to love those crispy bits. It didn't matter what food particularly but there's usually some crispy bits. Any sugars, refined carbs or meat so over-cooked as to be crispy or burnt gets converted in the process to being full of Advanced Glycation End-products. These AGEs (pun intended) are one of the primary drivers of physical ageing and decay.

If they ever invent those virtual holiday machines like they had in the movie 'Total Recall,' I will just stay where I am strapped into that chair and eat virtual crispy bits.

I own a soda stream machine – the classic 1970 design. I do not buy the syrups, I just make carbonated water. Harmless enough I thought. I'm still doing that because I like that effervescence in my mouth but now I know that all carbonated water contains phosphoric acid which reduced our body's ability to metabolise calcium. My fizzy tongue could be leading to brittle bones. You might want to check out a label on a bottle of coca-cola to see how much phosphoric acid it has. The acidity is offset by the massive amounts of sugar or sweeteners. And, in turn, the acidity stops the massive doses of sugar from making us vomit.

Osteoporosis is a major problem for older people but it starts well before anyone gets old. And it may not be that you're not getting enough calcium; it may be that the calcium you are getting isn't getting through. Osteoporosis may not be a calcium deficiency disease, it may be a disease of too much acidity. Acidity isn't just from soda, it's also from red meat. Bone fractures at whatever age for whatever duration set the stage for other problems down the line with their inherent immobility, inflammation and over-compensation.

Governments put out 'food pyramids' and other guides to the general population as to what we should be eating but these are no doubt influenced by food industry lobbyists. Besides, I've already warned you against generalised advice. Everyone's different and at different ages and given different circumstances, your needs fluctuate. Stay alert to what your body is telling you and take action on the feedback it is giving you.

More useful than one-size-fits-all pyramids are models like www.myplate.gov indicating portion controls. That has value. Our bodies cannot store protein. Adults only need 0.8g of protein per day per kilogram of body weight.

Remember those Nobel prize-winning Telomeres researchers? They recommend a bucket-load of expensive supplements, the more expensive of which they peddle themselves but they do also have a top 20 list of telomeres-friendly foods which are hard to argue with:

1. Blueberries

2. Grapefruit

3. Almonds

4. Apples

5. Avocados

6. Beetroot

7. Broccoli

8. Sweet potatoes

9. Garlic

10. Olive oil

11. Oranges

12. Wild salmon

13. Eggs

14. Tea

15. Tomatoes

16. Lean, non-processed meats

17. Beans

18. Sea vegetables

19. Cabbage

20. Kale

Of all the old wives' tales about healing foods and herbs, science seems to be consistently OK with the following:

- Garlic,

- Vinegar,

- Ginger,

- Green tea,

- Tumeric.

I'm not sure about vinegar. You may be supposed to soak your feet in it?

Sugar is a tough one. Most of us love sugar-based products and that is a primal driver. Things you didn't even know had sugar in them have sugar in them. One McDonalds cheeseburger has 7 grams of sugar in it. So does a Burger King cheeseburger. 7 grams of sugar is about 2 teaspoons. And who eats just one cheeseburger?

www.sugarstacks.com is a neat idea. I can say 7 grams but what does that look like? You might re-think drinking one can of coca cola if first you saw a photo of one can of coca cola with 10 sugar cubes next to it. Probably not, because you're addicted to sugar, but at least now you're operating from an informed position. If you're thinking that consuming 10 cubes of sugar would make you sick, you'd be correct but fortunately there are offsetting chemicals in soft drinks to enable us to consume and keep down the sugar.

It was once rumoured that cocaine was the secret ingredient in coca cola to addict drinkers to the product. No need. The World Health Organisation recommends no more sugar daily than:

Child	3tsp (12g)
Adult Female	5tsp (20g)
Adult Male	9tsp (36g)

And by sugar, they don't just mean the sweet powdery granules you add to tea or cereal. They also mean naturally occurring sugars like in fruit juice. In this sense, a 500ml container of Charlie's Real Orange Juice contains 11tsp of sugar – 22% more than a grown-as man's daily need. Of course, if you wanted to lose weight after a lifetime of excessive sugar consumption, you'd need to consume even less. New Zealanders are the 11th largest consumers of soft drinks in the world. On average we consume 10tsp of sugar daily *just from drinks*, nevermind however else we consume sugar. Six cans of coke a week at 139 calories per can, all other things being equal, will add five and a half kilograms to your weight in a year.

Fancy one of those ye olde branded fruit leathers you can get at a health store? Dehydrated fruits are 50% sugar - all of the sugars and nearly none of the nutrients. A cup of dried mangos has 76 grams of sugar. A mars bar has only 31 grams. Only!

The Otago Daily Times ran a story in April 2012 with the headline, **'Woman Drank 10 Litres Of Coke A Day Before Death.'** It's all very sad but especially her surviving partner's comments, "She drank at least 10 litres a day. As a family we would buy four 2.5 litres a day, the maximum on special. The Coke would be for Natasha to consume over the course of the day. The first thing she would do in the morning was have a drink of Coke and the last thing she would do in the day was have a drink of Coke by her bed... I never thought about it. It's just a soft drink, just like drinking water. I didn't think a soft drink was going to kill her."

The Coroner's medical expert, Dr Dan Mornin, told the court Harris probably had severe hypokalemia, a lack of potassium in the blood, relating to excessive consumption of soft-drinks. The main finding of death was from a cardiac arrhythmia.

It's easy to get super-judgemental here but selling soft drinks isn't inherently evil and consuming them isn't inherently stupid. That her partner thought 10 litres of Coke a day was harmless is a damning indictment of something; I'm just not entirely sure of what. Maybe the education system or a society increasingly devoid of personal responsibility?

The Coroner said although it was difficult to confirm this from post-mortem tests, it was consistent with her symptoms of tiredness and lack of strength and other cases of heavy soft-drink consumers, and it was likely her daily vomiting was due to too much caffeine, medically known as caffeine toxicity.

A study on rats by Connecticut College found that eating Oreo cookies activated more neurons in the brain's "pleasure centre" than exposure to cocaine or morphine. I look forward to seeing this in Oreo's advertising any day now. Perhaps it's less bad in you split them and lick out the filling first? Perhaps not?

Project leader Professor Joseph Schroeder says, "Our research supports the theory that high-fat, high-sugar foods stimulate the brain in the same way that drugs do." And like most humans, Schroeder says of the rats, "They don't seem to get much pleasure out of eating rice cakes." Buying cocaine is risky and expensive, whereas buying Oreos is not. How does Neuroscience student Jamie Honohan feel about Oreos after taking part in the research? "Now, I can't even look at them."

Feeling wholesome ordering your wraps? Check the ingredients in the three sauces you ask them to lash on. Except, of course, you either can't or won't. But, in your defence, you're probably not going to consume half a litre of sauce in a single sitting. At university, I saw that happen once during an orientation week. It did not end well.

In the form of juice, (and don't we all think juice is a 'good guy') we consume more sugars than we would normally. A box of orange juice we can drink easily. It might contain the sugar of five oranges. We probably wouldn't eat five oranges. Plus we don't get the fibre and several other benefits we would get from eating actual oranges.

Subway promotes itself as a healthier alternative. We now live in an age where a marketing position that is, effectively, the catch-cry, "We're less bad!" is considered virtuous. And it is. Of all the fast food places, they make a reasonable effort to put forward the nutritional information of their offerings. As opposed to the pizza companies who put it on the bottom of the boxes. You can't read it before you finish the pizza because the pizza will fall out and it's hard to read after because the grease has soaked through rendering the printing illegible. The latter may be a clue to the nutritional content of the offering.

Subway displays and promotes detailed nutritional information. This is to their credit and for this they wear a 'health halo.' A study by Brian Wansink assessed the recall of Subway customers versus McDonalds customers on nutritional information and their perceptions of how much they'd eaten, then compared their perception to how much they'd actually eaten. Three times as many Subway customers recalled seeing that there was some nutritional information but only a tiny fraction could recall specifics. All they remembered was that Subway displayed it. People tend to remember and perceive such things as black and white. It's either healthy or it is not. Our brains aren't into 'less bad': They like good and bad. Subway's display of nutritional information gives them a psychic tick and once there, most people order whatever they want cart blanche because 'everything' gets the mental tick.

Other research shows that only 9% of food purchasers look at the nutritional information generally and only 1% look beyond the headline 'total calories.' Health and productivity isn't so much about how many calories you eat, although that is important, it is mostly about *what* you eat. Not all calories are created equal. We don't have to eat like saints or sparrows. We do need to lessen our saturated fat and carbohydrate consumption and minimise sugars.

Yes, the McDonalds customers ate more and yes they estimated they ate 25% less calories than they actually did. Subway customers ate 35% more calories than they thought they did.

Eating sugar, or any of its sweetener alternatives regardless of how 'natural' they are, will drive spikes in your desire for more sweet things. Excessive consumption of refined sugars can lead to:

- Blocked cellular membranes resulting in slower neural communication (Duh!),

- Increased brain inflammation,

- Increase in the stress hormone cortisol, impairing memory,

- Impaired synaptic communication,

- Misfiring neurons and more of the slower alpha, delta and theta brainwaves leading to feelings of confusion.

Sugar intolerance looks like depression. Instead of taking Prozac, many people should stop taking M&Ms. So-called breakfast drink 'Up & Go' is described by their manufacturers as a "nutritious liquid breakfast" with "the protein, energy and dietary fibre of 2 Weet-Bix." How would they go in the Sugarstacks test? Nineteen grams in a 250ml pack! That's more than in a cheeseburger but only half that of a 355ml can of coke – a mere five sugarcubes. Their adverts feature young men drinking the product and their biceps bulging in an instant. They'd be a tad more honest if it was their gut doing the bulging.

I'm currently testing a new iPhone app called Foodswitch. Partly funded by a health insurer, it enables you to scan barcodes of food products in your pantry, or on the shelf at the supermarket, and it presents you with what its database considers to be healthier options. Often these are more 'less bad' than 'good' but, nevertheless, it's a small and helpful stepping stone to nudge people into making better (less bad) choices.

You know those sheets of seaweed used to roll up Sushi? Get some of those, spray them lightly with olive oil and bake them to create your own less unhealthy snack. If you absolutely have to eat cake, make it yourself and make it with friends or family.

Sugarstack's visual approach is effective, as are other influence strategies. Jeni Cross, a Sociologist at Colorado State University, speaks about a campaign in her State to encourage homeowners to insulate their houses. Education and publicity managed to get 20% of homeowner to insulate. The new campaign tripled that rate achieving a 60% insulation rate. What did they do?

Their presentations applied three approaches:

1. Tangibility
2. Personalised
3. Interactive

For example, instead of reporting to a homeowner that they had sixteen metres of gaps letting out expensive heat. They showed them what that looked like in total. It was a hole the equivalent size of a basketball. They knew what a basketball looked like and its scale. You knew what 7 grams is but it is a photo of a can of coke with 10 sugar cubes next to that has a dramatic and pragmatic effect on actual behaviour.

I have an initial personal aversion to what seems to be an increasingly international phenomenon – a sugar tax. A study published in the British Medical Journal said a 20 per cent tax on drinks with added sugar would decrease the number of obese adults by 1.3% and overweight adults by 0.9%. That seems a tiny reduction. I see problems with "added sugar" being the tax trigger. What about natural sugars? What about non-sugars that are essentially sugar? I applaud the sentiment but as usual such interventions end up being unfair and lumber a cost of compliance upon businesses. University of Otago Wellington public health researcher associate professor Nick Wilson says other things are needed, like food labelling and healthy school lunches.

Having gone largely sugar-free recently myself, I can attest to there being a lot more benefits that mere obesity reduction. That said, someone should probably do something, as Ministry of Health surveys have found more than one quarter of New Zealand adults aged 15 years and over, and one in 12 children, are obese. And that someone should be you. Forget about everyone else and society and worry about yourself and your loved ones. It's OK to worry a little bit. Long-living people worry just the right amount.

It's never too late to start reaping the benefits of wiser food choices, even if you can't 100% undo the effects of a lifetime of poor choices. A 2007 study at the Medical University of South Carolina looked at 15,000 people aged 45-64 years for 10 years. After 6 years, about 10% of the group started eating 'healthy.' Not dieting but eating healthy. They did reap better health and lower mortality. But diets sell because as the study's author put it, no one is going rush to buy a book whose slogan is, "Look slimmer in just six years."

> *"I bought a Christmas pudding that*
> *claimed to be sugar-free, gluten-free and*
> *dairy-free. I opened the box. It was a bowl of*
> *raisins." – Terry Williams, 'The Grin Reaper'*
> *comedy show*

In 2000, Cornell University's Brian Wansink, author of the book 'Mindless Eating', ran a test on movie goers. They all got free tubs of popcorn. Half got a massive sized tub and the other half got an even more massive tub. All the popcorn had been deliberately aged and made stale. The containers were assessed to see how much had been eaten. Even though the 'food' itself was gross and no rational person should have eaten anything, those people with the bigger tubs ate 53% more. Society and governments try to promote healthy eating through education and those methods are proving ineffective as Jeni Gross highlighted earlier. Chip and Dan Heath in their book 'Switch' argue that the solution needs to be practical, specific and direct. The solution isn't about educating the eaters; the solution is smaller tubs.

Satirical news website 'The Onion' ran a delightfully cutting yet disturbingly prescient item on the crowds protesting the Mayor of New York's proposed ban on the sale of sweetened beverages larger than 16 ounces. "While many argue that people in this country lack the passion and general informedness to meaningfully participate in matters of public policy, the fierce outcry against the soda ban provides depressing evidence that this is not entirely true. This embarrassingly powerful demonstration of democracy shows that, when their backs are against the wall, Americans are unfortunately still very willing to band together and stand up for what they believe in most. Specifically, soda." The article goes on to note the lack of demonstrations against drone strikes on civilians.

Wansink has run some fun experiments proving how big containers, plates and packaging affect our consumption. He's used magic 'bottomless' soup bowls to show that people keep on eating. With trick technology covertly pumping more soup into bowls as they ate, diners consumed 73% more than diners with a non-trick plate who could go back for more. Give people a 34oz bowl instead of a 17oz bowl and they'll eat 31% more. It's not about how full our tummies are but how full our plates still are. Wansink also found that people drink 30% less out of tall, thin glasses than short wide ones. People offered a pound bag of M&Ms eat 137 on average, whereas people offered a half pound bag eat 71 on average.

But if we interrupt the patterns that make it easy for us to continue eating, we're quite capable of doing so. Observing people given containers of potato chips where every 10th one was coloured red, many more stopped after 10 than where all the chips were indistinguishable. How can we programme in our own 'stop signs'?

We overeat for a number of reasons – plate or glass size, packaging, bulk buying and worrying about waste, and distractions. Distractions are a real problem. TV itself is not an inherently bad thing but these are bad things:

- Being alone

- Remaining motionless

- Eating mindlessly

TV habitualises all those things. Let's not look at remote villages with wonderfully healthy traditions. Let's look at a study of Americans who lost weight and managed to keep it off. What common factors did they have?

- 92% exercised at home,

- 78% ate breakfast every day,

- 75% weighed themselves at least once a week,

- They averaged TV watching of less than ten hours a week.

Getting vitamins via food has benefits that don't occur when those same vitamins are taken in the form of supplements or even juice. There are other enzymes and fibre in food that help the digestion, processing and absorption of the vitamins. Microbes in your gut aid in food digestion and synthesising vitamins. These microbes vary from person to person and we may all be 'colonised' by a particular strain of them early in our lives. There are a few major classifications, similar to how blood types are classified. Knocking back a probiotic yoghurt from the supermarket is a good thing but would be a better thing if we knew our type and could match it to the right yoghurt.

Probiotics are of growing interest in health care for their potential in helping to treat a number of conditions, including irritable bowel syndrome, tooth decay and chronic fatigue syndrome. The Wall Street Journal reported that, for all their infection-fighting power, antibiotics kill the good bugs along with the bad in the intestine. The result is an imbalance in the gut that can lead a bacterium known as Clostridium difficile— C. diff for short—to colonize and produce a toxin that can cause diarrhea, dehydration and fever. In severe cases, C. diff infections can lead to kidney failure, recurrent infection and death. Analyses by researchers at Maimonides Medical Centre in Brooklyn, N.Y., in 2011 found that using probiotics for periods ranging from a few days to three weeks reduced a patient's odds of developing antibiotic-associated diarrhea by 60%. So, even if you don't live longer, the life you lead will be less gross than it would have been otherwise. They say there's no such thing as a free lunch but perhaps in future, via the public health system, you might be able to score some free yoghurt. Mind you, if you were a yoghurt fan, you'd be less likely to be in the hospital in the first place, right?

There may even be a 'Brain – Gut' connectivity that affects our emotions, sense of well-being and feelings. Tell me you've never received some bad news and experienced a sinking sensation *in your gut*. Well, it goes both ways.

Freshly frozen foods from your supermarket can be more nutritious than so-called fresh foods in the same stores that have travelled a bit. Vegetables and fish especially get snap frozen before much nutritional loss occurs.

Lincoln Tan from the NZ Herald reported on research from the University of Sydney's Charles Perkins Centre. They found the instinctive appetite for protein in humans is so powerful, people continue to eat until their bodies get the right amount of protein. The overriding drive for dietary protein was a core factor in the global obesity epidemic, especially as diets shifted towards an increased proportion of foods higher in carbohydrates and fats and with protein reduced.

"We found that regardless of your age or body mass index, your appetite for protein is so strong that you will keep eating until you get enough protein, which could mean eating much more than you should," said lead author Dr Alison Gosby. Most people tend to eat the right amount of protein but they eat way too much in order to get to that point.

Get some eggs into you for breakfast I reckon. As many as you can place in one of your hand open flat without rolling off. If one rolls off, don't eat that egg. In fact, you'd better grab some paper towels with your spare hand. (I probably should have told you that first.) You will eat less dross throughout the day with a great protein-laden start like that.

In Dan Buettner's Blue Zone of Okinawa, the locals have a saying, "Hara Hachi Bu." This means to eat until you're not hungry as opposed to eating until you're full. There's a time lag between satiating our appetite and our brains making us feel full. Eat til you're 80% full and you'll be about right. If there's food in front of you or within easy reach, especially trashy food, you'll eat more. Don't rely on willpower and being virtuous or having your own best interests at heart. Rely on only having real food, then only preparing enough.

Serve and put the rest away *before you eat* if there are left-overs. Make it *look* bigger; Use smaller plates. Make snacking a hassle. Buy smaller packages. Place obvious and regular reminders of why you don't want to become obese. Eat slow. Focus on the food itself not TV or other distractions. Sit down. Eat early.

One research effort looked at the impact of having evidence of what we've already eaten left in front of us on how much more we choose to eat. The study used chicken wings at a Super Bowl party. Waiting staff only bussed the bones off of half of the tables. The group with the bony evidence in front of them ate 28% less. If you think restaurants and cafes bus your tables for your comfort and to look tidy, think again. If there's no evidence in front of you that you've eaten, you feel hungrier and are more likely to order more food. The same goes for bars and bottles. Try keeping the caps off the bottles of beer you order in a bar and see how that works. Most will pre-remove the caps 'for your convenience.' The same goes for topping up wine glasses.

Our stomachs and digestive system do have their own fairly independent nervous system but it's pretty stupid and has a terrible memory. It takes twenty minutes from when our stomach gets to a satiated state before that signal hits our brains but how often do we allow ourselves the opportunity to receive that twenty minute signal?

Meal Type	*Average Duration*
Fast food outlet (alone)	11 minutes
Workplace cafeteria (alone)	13 minutes
Medium restaurant (alone)	28 minutes
Medium Restaurant (with 3 others)	56 minutes

"The ice cream company making Magnum ice creams did its research. People felt guilty eating luxury ice creams on a stick. So they came up with the new Mini-Magnum – half the size and half the calories... only available in packs of six." – Terry Williams, 'The Grin Reaper' comedy show

So much of what is marketed as food might better be described as 'edible substances.' You'd be smart not to eat anything that had been processed so much that it is more a product of industry than nature. Here are some general tips that you know you already know:

- Don't eat anything that your grandmother wouldn't recognise as food,

- Don't eat anything that is incapable of decomposing,

- Don't eat anything containing ingredients that are unfamiliar, unpronounceable, or are more than 5 in number. Nothing good for you has 6 ingredients,

- Beware 'ticks' from organisations like a 'heart tick.' They over-focus. A low-fat product might get a tick but if it's laden with sugar, that's as bad for your heart as fat,

- Unless you have to, try and avoid getting fuel for yourself from the same place that you get fuel for your car,

- Organic does not necessarily equate to healthy. They can produce organic high fructose corn syrup. It's better for nature, it is not better for you.

The people who want you to buy their foodlike substances have more money and time than you, and they've been experimenting on us for us years, not just in production but marketing. Full credit to their scientists. Tomato sauce or ketchup is a great case in point.

Us humans have five basic tastes: salty, bitter, sour, sweet and umami. Umami is a full-bodies proteinish taste we first experienced via mother's milk. Modern tomato sauce is a pretty decent delivery system for tomato concentrate which may well prove to lower the odds of men getting prostate cancer. But it delivers others things as well. Check out the sugar content.

Taste is there to tell our bodies about the food we're eating. We're very attracted to sweetness because in nature very few sweet tasting things can kill us. The umami flavouring makes our bodies believe we're getting vital protein intake and we are not. I wrote a few pages ago of our drive for protein and how we eat too much overall to get our protein. Our sauces are contributing to our over-consumption. It's more the fault of sauces manufactured by scientists rather than those made by your grandmother.

Brian Wansink, who ran so many entertaining and enlightening studies on how we eat without thinking, suggests three eating re-engineering strategies:

1. Don't aim to eat like a tri-athlete monk. Simply aim to eat 20% less overall and 20% more vegetables,

2. Food visibility – hide the sweet stuff and display the healthy and natural stuff (Office workers given jars of candy ate 71% less when those jars were not see-through),

3. 'Table-scaping' – smaller plates, plates with a colour that clashes with the food colour, putting away leftovers before eating, etc

The more hassle it is to eat, the less we eat. Design your schedule and environment so it's logistically easier to eat more vegetables. Be wary of buying bulk deals to save money. People eat stockpiled food at twice the normal rate.

Eat on a regular schedule. If your body is expecting lunch and you miss it, you don't just feel hungry or listless. Cortisol gets released into your bloodstream to thicken your blood, conserve energy and preserve fat. Our bodies like homeostasis and if you don't maintain it, your body will. Our balance of hormones is sorted out while we sleep. The consequences of poor sleep go way beyond feeling tired the next day.

"I wish I hated pizza as much as it hates me." – Jim Gaffigan

5.3.1.3

Sleep

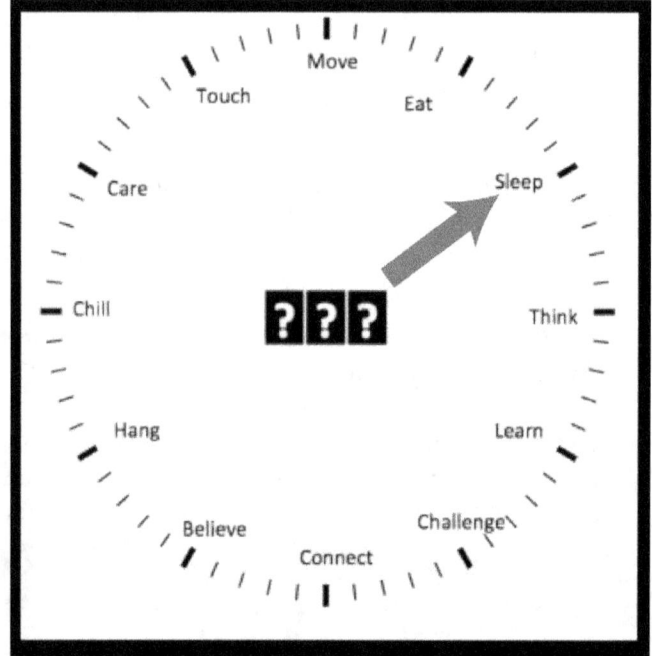

Poor sleep can increase stroke risk 400%,

Ineffective sleep makes you immediately less productive,

Poor sleep heightens risk of dementia & makes you a pain to be around.

Mark Wolverton wrote in *Psychology Today* of a seminal 2002 study that revealed a strong relationship between an individual's reported sleep and mortality. "People who slept less than seven hours a night—or more than nine—were at increased risk for all-cause mortality," says University of Pittsburgh psychiatrist Martica Hall. Other studies revealed a similar curvilinear relationship between sleep duration and conditions such as cardiovascular disease and obesity.

Your body's 'Circadian Clock' broadly follows the expected natural patterns of night and day with your brain and cells attentive to external cues such as temperature, sounds and light. Modern life and your behaviour messes with those natural cues to varying degrees at varying times. Plus we consume things like caffeine and alcohol. If you poured coffee, Red Bull or Jack Daniels into your TiVo, it would probably struggle to record 'The Walking Dead' at the right time for you. Your body reacts much the same way.

Research from the University of Surrey published earlier this year helps explain how insufficient sleep alters gene expression - offering important clues to the ways in which sleep and health are linked at the molecular level. The study's authors found that after a single week of insufficient sleep (fewer than six hours nightly) blood samples from participants revealed altered activity in over 700 genes, including those related to heart disease, diabetes, metabolism, and inflammatory, immune, and stress responses.

Sleep is an essential restorative function, in more ways than one. But for a start, here's just one way reported in Forbes by Melanie Heiken. When you sleep, your brain undergoes a cleaning process that removes waste linked to Alzheimer's and Dementia, according to a study by the University of Rochester Medical Centre. They used imaging to look deep into the brains of mice and observed that the brain functions differently while asleep, mopping up accumulated proteins at a much faster rate. Led by Maiken Nedergaard, the researchers discovered that a waste-draining system they call the 'Glymphatic System' is ten times more active during sleep than while awake. This nocturnal cleaning system removes proteins called amyloid-beta, which accumulate into the plaques that may contribute to Alzheimer's disease and Dementia.

Researchers at the Erasmus MC University Medical Center in Rotterdam, the Netherlands, and the University of Surrey in the UK measured white blood cell counts in young men who sleep eight hours and men whose sleep was restricted, and found a spike in white blood cells, particularly those called granulocytes, released in response to immune system threat. So it would seem that severe sleep loss jolts the immune system just as stress does and, if that accumulates, it affects your health. It could quadruple your risk of a stroke. Though researchers don't know the exact mechanism, it seems that chronic lack of sleep causes inflammation, elevates blood pressure and heart rate, and affects glucose levels, leading to a much higher stroke risk in the sleep-deprived.

Sleep increases the ability of the four main healthy lifestyle habits (a healthy diet, exercise, moderate alcohol consumption and not smoking) to protect the body against cardiovascular disease.

Good Sleep	*Without*	*With*
Cardio-Vascular Disease	Down 57%	Down 65%
Fatal Cardio-Vascular Disease	Down 67%	Down 83%

A study by the Harvard Medical School found that disrupted sleep patterns and irregular routines caused glucose self regulation in subjects to "go haywire." Even a lie-in contributes to that. U.K. researchers Yvonne Harrison and James Horne reviewed multiple studies on the impact of sleep deprivation on decision making and problem solving. They concluded that it can lead to impaired communication, a lack of flexibility and willingness to try alternatives, a reduced ability to innovate, and an inability to deal with rapidly changing situations. Poor sleep leads to poorer decision-making and, often, one of those poorer decisions is to not do anything about the poor sleep. Most people are blissfully unaware of how impaired they are with even minor levels of sleep disruption, nevermind those who think they can rock on after pulling an all-nighter.

Those heroic doctors and residents in hospitals working those famously long hours of theirs - a study in the *Archives of Surgery* found that residents were critically impaired by tiredness during more than a quarter of waking hours and that, when sleep deprived, they were 22% more likely to commit medical errors. A 2009 JAMA study revealed an increased rate of complications when surgical procedures were performed by Doctors who had less than a six-hour window for sleep between their last procedure the day before and the first procedure the next day.

Poor sleep affects us mentally and physically in all spheres of our life. Once again, it's utterly interconnected and can spiral if we're not careful. We don't need to be puritan about it, just sensible. Easier said than done it seems for many.

When asked about the best tool to sort out poor sleep, sleep researcher Brad Cardinal responded, "Regular physical activity is better than any meds."

Sheldon Cohen's researchers at Carnegie Mellon University tested sleep and immunity. They exposed healthy adults to cold viruses, isolating and monitoring for five days afterwards. People who had been recently under stress showed increased resistance to Cortisol. They also found participants had more Cytokines, which trigger inflammation.

In their book 'NutureShock', Po Bronson and Ashley Merryman detail how sleep impacts our attitude. Negative stimuli get processed by the amygdala. Positive or neutral stimuli get processed by the hippocampus. Lack of sleep affects the hippocampus more than it does the amygdala. Therefore, sleep-deprived people struggle to recall pleasant memories but remember downcast ones well. In a word-memorising study, sleep-deprived participants could remember 81% of negative words such as 'cancer', yet only 31% of positive or neutral ones like 'basket' or 'sunshine.'

So what does it all mean? That when you get stressed out and stop sleeping, or stop sleeping well, you get sick. So, poor sleep can lead to dementia, stroke, depression and lowered immunity to illness generally – all of which feeds on itself in a negative spiral. How much sleep should you get and how can you improve your odds of getting that?

Soft ear plugs, eye shades, routine, listen to white noise, no caffeine or alcohol.

For most people, the best sleep duration is seven hours. Those averaging eight hours have 12% worse morbidity than those sleeping seven. From a longevity point of view, it would be better to sleep five hours than eight. "People who slept less than seven hours a night - or more than nine - were at increased risk for all-cause mortality," says University of Pittsburgh psychiatrist Martica Hall.

A sleep-supportive evening meal would not be too late and would consist of complex carbs, magnesium and protein. Examples are chicken with broccoli with a low-fat cheese sauce or a cheese and vegetable pasta. Chuck in some spinach or kale for the magnesium. Other options include dark leafy greens, pumpkin seeds, mackerel, tuna, beans, brown rice, avocado, plain yoghurt, bananas, figs, or dark chocolate. Don't eat less than two hours before sleeping and keep night-time meals light on the spices.

Decent vegetable sources of protein are:

- Asparagus,

- Avocado,

- Beans,

- Broccoli,

- Cauliflower,
- Chickpeas,
- Lentils,
- Peas,
- Quinoa,
- Spinach,
- Almonds,
- Cashews,
- Peanuts,
- Peas,
- Pistachios,
- Walnuts.

If Marie Antoinette was alive today and made aware of the grumblings of the peasants, she might exclaim, "Let them eat quinoa."

Various studies propose a range of tips:

- Be consistent,
- Have a routine,
- Empty your mind,
- Before bed, avoid alcohol, caffeine, nicotine or a big meal,
- Exercise earlier in the day,
- Block out stimuli,
- Seek snoring solutions,
- Don't be obese,

- Check your mattress and pillow.

Make your bedroom a couple of degrees cooler than the rest of your house, irrespective of the season. Darken your rooms the hour before your bedtime. Light affects our melatonin levels and that's a big player in sleep. The light from TVs and smartphones will mess with that. Smartphone screen illumination can suppress melatonin production by 20%. It is bad enough that you'll fret about some email you checked when you didn't have to at 11pm but that light smacking your eyeballs will make it worse. It may be that the electronic paper screens of eReaders do not have the same negative effect.

One app that adjusts the light emanating from your device is 'f.lux.' It knows what time it is where you are and what the natural light levels should be. It knows that your eyes should be receiving signals from that environmental light to synch up with your biology for, amongst other things, our sleep cycle. With that knowledge, it filters and adjusts the light type and levels to suit. Computer screens, tablets and mobile phones emit full spectrum light around the clock, just like the sun. Exposure to blue light at the wrong time of day can keep you awake later and interfere with the quality of your sleep. f.lux tries to help this by removing blue and green light to help you wind down in the evenings. At the time of writing, they've had 8 million downloads.

I have another iPhone app called 'Sleep Cycle' which monitors my body movements as I sleep and works out where in the sleep cycle of my circadian rhythms I am at. I might set the alarm for 6am but it can unilaterally wake me at 5:47 if that is the optimum time closest to 6am for my brain's cycles. No doubt there are other products. I can't swear for the science behind it but when I'm having trouble sleeping, usually during periods of extensive travel where all the exercise, eating and stress patterns go out the door, I find it helpful.

Live, Work, Love

It may actually exist for real now but I saw a single-frame cartoon of an iPhone alarm clock app with the snooze button costing you $1.99. It's funny, but with a real seed of truth about it.

> *"Sleep is a waste of time." – Thomas Edison (Inventor of the lightbulb, possibly the single item most responsible for messing up our Circadian Rhythms.)*

5.3.2

Mental

I tend to pick and choose the digestible chunks from writers that might be labelled as alternative, holistic or new age. Or hippy freaks. So, I'm a bit of an eye-roller when Deepak Chopra writes, "Although each person seems separate and independent, all of us are connected to patterns of intelligence that govern the whole cosmos." Does the universe and everything in it vibrate at different frequencies and if only you can think thoughts about what you want, you'll tune in via those frequencies and make your dreams come true. I think not. Thinking about what you want, by itself, won't get you what you want. There's increasing evidence that it's counter-productive.

That's my disclaimer and cynicism about new age holistic writings. But what was once loopy, gains credibility once evidence is gathered via the scientific process. So, when Deepak Chopra writes, "The biochemistry of the body is a product of awareness. Beliefs, thoughts and emotions create the chemical reactions that uphold life in every cell. An aging cell is the end product of awareness that has forgotten how to remain new." This concept I can buy into – the psychology-physiology connection. I don't think you can think yourself young again. But the next four Mental controls are about how you can control your state of mind and that state of mind is a major driver of your health, wellbeing, productivity and longevity.

Childhood or lifetime habits of being happy, popular, outgoing, taking it easy, playing it safe or avoiding stress generally do not lead to a long and healthy life.

Lewis Terman began a study that would outlast even himself. From 1921 to 2001, his Stanford University study looked at 1528 participants and found out the extent to which our childhood traits impacted the rest of our lives. I'm no fan of studies that use self reporting. Who knows how honest people are about what they think they remember they felt about what they might have done? Terman's study was observational and detailed and looong.

Using the five-factor CANOE model of personality (Conscientiousness, Agreeableness, Neuroticism, Openness, Extroversion), they found that those people with lifelong conscientiousness fared best in the lifespan stakes. Conscientious people tend to be thrifty, persistent, detail-oriented and responsible. This means they tend to do more things that protect their health and engage in fewer risky activities. They lead themselves into healthier situations and relationships. With conscientiousness as a predictor, they create healthy, lifelong pathways for themselves.

Terman was a Eugenicist and super racist so I'm never going to be a big fan of him but this study raises some interesting and non-repugnant points.

We can choose to change. We don't have to be as were as children and this study showed that many people did vary their traits over time and that this did impact their lifespan and health.

As a child As	*Premature death*	Conscientious	Conscientious	Not conscientious	Not conscientious
		Conscientious	Not conscientious	Conscientious	Not conscientious
		Lowest risk	Low risk	Medium risk	

a				Hig
n				h
a				risk
d				
u				
l				
t				

A 1990 study at Yale by Horwitz et al looked at heart attack sufferers and their adherence to treatment. So these were people who had ***just had a heart attack*** – how much bigger a wake-up call do you need? The non-conscientious personalities took less than 75% of their meds and were 200% more likely to die within a year. That risk was equally as true for those on placebos! Conscientiousness doesn't just make you a good person, it makes you a healthy and long-living person.

Even when conscientious people get pushed off their path by external events, they are far more likely to get back on. They have good friends, are involved with others in a consequential life, find a happy relationship, persistently achieve via hard work plus meaning and purpose, take charge of their thoughts, do not catastrophise, are resilient and do a moderate amount of worrying.

Between 1996 and 2006, the rate of people seeking psychotherapy in the US rose 150%. A study at the Department of Cardiology at the University of Heidelberg looked at the incidence of pre-operative depression in patients undergoing surgery due to narrowing of the blood vessels feeding the heart. They developed a psychology testing model that predicts with 90% accuracy the risk of death during surgery. Another study found that after we experience the bereavement of a loved one or immediate family member (not always the same thing), our risks go up for diabetes, ulcerative colitis, TB, glaucoma and gum abscesses. Our state of mind affects our body's state.

5.3.2.1

Think

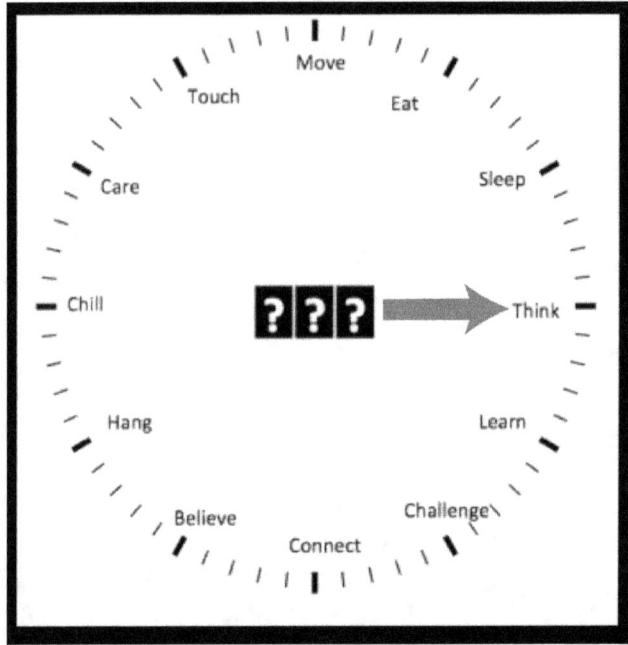

You can make big improvements in your life with small changes,

Overly stressful thinking over time causes physical damage,

Focus drives behaviour.

Psychoneuroimmunology (PNI) is the study of the interaction between psychological processes and the nervous and immune systems of the human body. The main interests of PNI are the interactions between the nervous and immune systems and the relationships between mental processes and health.

In 1979, Ellen Langer, now Professor of psychology at Harvard, ran what became known as the 'Counter-clockwise Study.' She set up a residence that was completely outfitted as if it was 1959. She got in a group of subjects in their late 70s and early 80s and pre-tested them on weight, dexterity, flexibility, vision, taste sensitivity, IQ, visual memory, appearance and ran a psychological self-evaluation. The subjects spent a week in 1979 living as if it was back in 1959, immersed in things and thoughts from that time. They were not even allowed to discuss events that occurred after that year and were to encourage each other not to do so. Their clothes, the food, the radio, TV, sports, news allowed in the residence were all from 1959.

The subjects were then post-tested across the same criteria with marked improvements on all of them. On top of the measurements, they stood taller, walked faster and spoke more confidently. Even if these were temporary effects, there are positive physical consequences for standing straight for your spine, airways and digestion. Confidence can boost your social life which, again, boosts longevity and quality of life. All these factors work together but they start with our mental state. Such is the sway of our thinking on our physiology.

Such is the power of possibilities. It certainly puts a new spin on the old saying, "Act Your Age!"

The brain accounts for two percent of your body's weight yet consumes 50% of your oxygen and 25% of your energy. Brain cells don't die of old age but they do shrink, thus the distance between connections increases lowering efficiency. However, connections between neurons can increase and be stimulated to do so.

A University of Michigan study showed that a 1% increase in optimism (albeit self-rated) corresponded to a 9% decrease in the incidence of stroke.

A University of Texas study showed that journaling improves immunity. A record of life, expressing emotions that otherwise may have gone repressed, collecting goals, plans and new ideas.

Ellen Langer ran a study of people and what they wore and its impact on health. She compared people who wore uniforms to those that didn't in comparable income brackets. Morbidity data was assessed from 1986 to 1994 across 206 professions. The thinking was that uniforms are ageless, whereas people who dressed as they were expected to for their age, might actually be made to feel their age due to how they dressed. The uniform wearers missed fewer work days, had fewer hospitalisations and contracted fewer chronic diseases. Author Catherine Mayer noted, "It's healthier to be mutton dressed as lamb than mutton dressed as mutton."

Clothing is an 'age cue.' Uniforms prevent clothing being an age cue because everyone in those jobs dresses the same regardless of age. What other age cues do you recognise? There might be baldness (rightly or wrongly), greying of hair or the expanding gut. It makes for an interesting observation of couples where there is a significant age difference. Do the cues from one affect the other? Does the young 'un age up and the old 'un age down, psychologically primed by the cues given out by the other? There are exceptions but, on average, yes they do.

In 1961, Yale Psychologist Neal Miller suggested that the autonomous nervous system that controls blood pressure and heart rate, without our conscious awareness, could be controlled and trained using our voluntary system, the same system I'm using to type these words. Subsequent studies found this to be possible with biofeedback via monitors.

On a broader level, for this to work we need feedback. We need to be alert for how we are. We need to be literally

'M*indful.*' Mindfulness is a state of active, open attention on the present. When you're mindful, you observe your thoughts and feelings from a distance, without judging them good or bad. Instead of letting your life pass you by, mindfulness means living in the moment and awakening to experience.

As you move towards greater Mindfulness, you'll notice the triggers that affect your physical and mental states, both positively and negatively. Armed with this information, you'll be much better positioned to make effective and lasting changes. Rather than generalised advice for random people that aren't you that you shouldn't eat cheese, you can make your own decisions based on your own data. Try things and see what happens. Do one thing wholeheartedly and with focus, like minimising your sugar intake for a month. Be open-minded and see what happens. Write your responses down and spot the trend.

Being Mindful is made harder and distorted by our inherent biases and prejudices. If you're reading this and thinking to yourself, 'I don't have any biases or prejudices," well, that's one of your biases and prejudices. As Anais Nin said, "We don't see things as they are, we see things are we are..."

One such bias is how we view exercise. This is one connection between the mental and the physical. Bias is kind of a judgemental label. Let's call it a mental model or a lens through which we view the world. Such lenses not only filter and distort how we perceive what we observe and experience, it affects the feedback we receive that drives our behaviours. Our parents, our lives and our decisions have shaped, polished or scratched our lenses but we can, of course, choose to change lenses any time we wish. But we have to want to.

Here's an example of how mental models affected people's behaviour and even their physiology. Ali Crum and Ellen Langer ran a trial with hotel cleaners. Generally, pre-testing showed that they had poor levels of health. Two thirds self-reported they did "no regular exercise" and one third self-reported they did "no regular exercise." They did not perceive via their mental models that the work they did each day was, itself, exercise. Analysis of the vacuuming, dusting, washing, bed-making and so forth showed it added up to as much as most people would achieve in a very vigorous gym session.

Half the cleaners were told of this and were given a brief educational session on the health benefits of the work activities they performed that were akin to exercise. The other half of the cleaners were not told. Both groups received pre measurements on weight, body fat, body water and blood pressure.

Four weeks later, post measurements revealed that the group educated on the value of exercise and that their work was akin to exercise had improved across the board. They'd lost weight, lost body fat percentage, gained body water percentage indicating increased muscle growth and lowered blood pressure. It'd be facetious to suggest that we can all 'think ourselves thin' but undoubtedly we can leverage our exercise by our attitudes which all starts from education and our mental models.

Catch and correct yourself in unhelpful and unhealthy thinking. Do you use absolutes such as "always" and "never"? Challenge them! Find evidence to the contrary. If you have a negative inner critical voice, it's impossible to ignore it and trying to will just draw your attention to it and give it unhelpful focus. This is a novel and surprisingly effective technique I've used myself and highly recommend. You can't stop the voice but adapt it. Convert it into the voice of a drunken loudmouth who shouts the words to you from the street below your window. You wouldn't pay attention to the obnoxious blathering from an actual wino in the street and, soon enough, you'll hold your inner critic in contemptuous disdain. I laughed at this but it really works. Your inner critic is a dickhead. Make them sound like one.

This inner critic is of course, different from your own inner monologue giving useful advice like, "Did I close the garage door? Better go back and check," or "Spending $200 on miracle weed superfood ointment is probably a waste of money and might actually harm me." This voice you should listen to and work with.

And once you've sidelined your inner dickhead, you need to replace that commentary with a deliberately chosen one of your own. Not useless and vague positive affirmations but clear and explicit goal-aligned replacement thoughts. Again looking at maintaining a healthy diet and the power of our thoughts in driving our behaviours, the U.S. National Weight Loss Control Registry Database looked at over 10,000 weight loss maintainers. Not only did they lose thirty or more pounds, they kept it off for at least a year at the time of surveying. What was their advice? Control your focus! Research healthy food ideas and fun physical activities as a hobby. The number one idea combining both was to plan and start a garden.

'Shoulds' are a bugbear to me personally. If you want to rile me, tell me I *should* do something. Don't give me a reason, just tell me I *should*. Shoulds will trick you. One study asked two groups to do jumping jacks. One group got asked to do 100 and the other 200. Both got tired two thirds of the way through. That's when most people think they should get tired.

Focus on what you want and not on what you're trying to avoid. Think about the words you use or are used on you. Cure versus remission, recovering versus recovered, supplements versus meds. Beware of labels like 'patient.'

Here are some negativity Traps:

- If it's not black, it must be white,

- If it's not perfect, it's no good,

- Why is this always happening to me?

- I'm not going to like this,

- I feel it so it must be true,

- I'm a label, you're a different label,

- I should do this, you should do that,

- If it's wrong, it must be my fault.

Daniel Wegner's studies showed us that it is hard to not think of something you don't wish to think about. In my last book 'The Brain-Based Boss', I cited his work:

Dan Wegner asked a class to think of anything except polar bears but if they should happen to think of a polar bear then they should ring a little bell he'd given to each of them. The classroom's airwaves were awash with ringing within seconds. This effect is called 'Ironic Reversal'. Variations on this study have been conducted over the years proving that if you want someone not to panic then the worst thing you can say is, "Don't panic." You'd be better off saying something like, "Remain calm". Saying, "Don't spill the milk," to a child or, "Don't look down," to a trainee tightrope walker would be equally counter-productive. And being counter-productive is something they teach you to avoid at tightrope-walking school.

This is especially true of emotion-laden negative thoughts. Some researchers suggest negative thought replacement. Like anything habitual, you can't just stop and leave a vacuum.

In his book 'Smarter Than You Think', Clive Thompson proposes some lessons on how we can improve our thinking. He uses the term "Cognitive Diversity" which means to me simply doing different things. The very existence of novelty in our lives stimulates our brains into creativity and interest. Back in caveman times, novelty was a threat – new things could eat you or be poisonous. These days, that's much less true. A survey of executives showed that their best new ideas came whilst travelling. I worked once with an advertising high-flyer who told me that when he managed their London office, they had a map of London on the wall. Every time they got a campaign got sign-off, they put a pin in the map marking the location of the idea originator at the moment they had their inspiration. Only ten percent of the pins were stuck into the office's location. The leading location was across the road in the pub but that's probably not the point here. Alcohol and sociability certainly play their part but it is the sameness of the office that sucks the creativity out of it. Non-changing locations and routines lacks cognitive diversity.

He uses another term – 'Cognitive Amplification.' This is when we take our original ponderings and put the out into the world. This might be as simple as passing a piece of note paper to another individual or posting a tweet on Twitter. More usefully, it is probably sharing your thinking with friends or colleagues, creating a feedback loop or spiral that edits the idea, feeding on the wisdom of crowds. Once again, social connections improve things, not only our health and longevity but the quality of our thinking. That is, of course, highly dependent on the quality of your connections. They don't have to be Einsteins but it would help if they were honest, good listeners and challenging. It is up to each of us to bolster and expand the quality of social and professional connections for many reasons. If nothing else, they are people to sell the fundraising chocolates and raffle tickets your kids bring home from school and sports clubs.

I do have to stop and check myself every time I use the term 'wisdom of crowds.' You've got to choose your crowds very carefully. On the homepage of most newspaper's websites you'll easily find a highly visible section listing their most popular headlines – those that have been clicked on the most. It's often a celebrity sighting or a royal baby. It's never the signing of a treaty for world peace. The day that I'm writing this sentence, my local paper's most popular news link is, and I quote, "Doctor Murray held Michael Jackson's penis every night." You've got to choose your crowds very carefully. (And your doctors too!)

Dr David Lykken's study showed that people have a happiness 'set point' to which we return eventually, regardless of what external circumstances are doing to us. Whether we're winning lotteries or burying loved ones, we hover around our own personal happiness level. And Lykken says that level is set genetically. Lykken was the proponent of a set-point theory of happiness, which argues that one's sense of well-being is half determined by genetics and half determined by circumstances. His research findings suggest that a person's baseline levels of cheerfulness, contentment, and psychological satisfaction are largely a matter of heredity. Lykken's advice was to seek a "steady diet of simple pleasures."I should also point out that Lykken proposed that Governments should licence people to become parents before they were legally allowed to have a baby. Probably best if we just do the simple pleasures thing for now.

Optimism is great but over-optimism is not, according to Terman's longitudinal study. Overly cheerful and optimistic children were less likely to live to an old age than their staid and sober counterparts. Over-optimism was a comparable risk to high blood pressure or high cholesterol. New Zealand culture has a catchphrase, "She'll be right," promoting a "Don't worry, be happy" lassez faire approach. It doesn't work. Realistic worrying is healthy, catastrophising is not.

With happiness, lasting adjustment occurs with smaller, progressive steps. It's like weight training in that regard. Watch less TV and only the good stuff. Improve your social relations. Increase your physical activity. Help others and express gratitude. Take on new challenges. It's all one great big inter-connected smorgasbord. But the smartest finding of all is that happiness does not lead to healthiness. Healthiness leads to happiness.

Live, Work, Love

"I didn't worry about other people's ability to spell until my cleaner sent me an invoice that included a charge for 'moping'."
– Terry Williams, 'The Grin Reaper' comedy show

5.3.2.2

Learn (Teach)

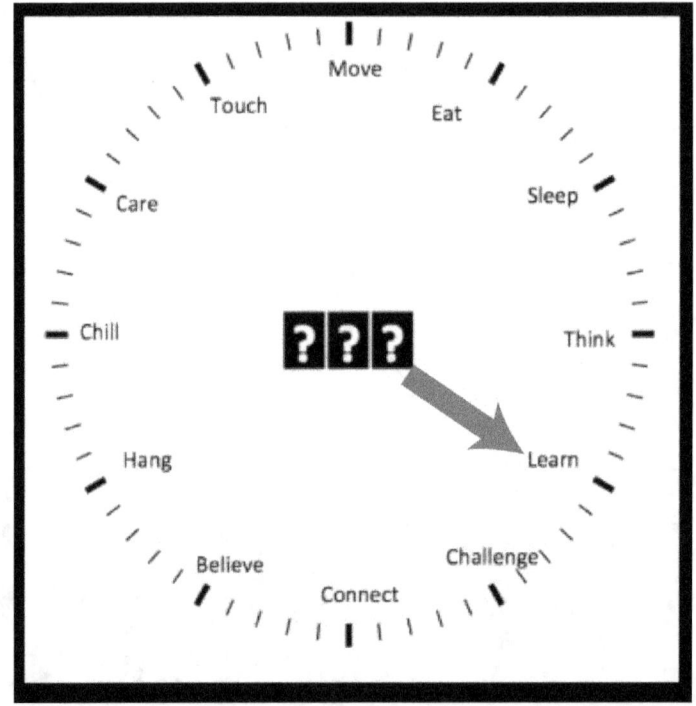

Ongoing mental stimulation lessens brain deterioration,

Social connections made through learning improve your odds,

Improved skills and knowledge make you matter more.

Maybe learning Spanish at age 50 won't prevent you from getting Dementia. Even if it doesn't, won't the attempt improve the quality of your life? Actually, bilingual people do have lower levels of dementia. They also have greater job security, better historical familial connections if they're immigrants, and higher remuneration. It's one of my minor life disappointments to work on soon that I do not have a smattering a few other languages. Just enough to start or stop a fight.

I initially pencilled in 'Learn' as a life enhancing control because I thought it would stimulate our minds in a physical sense and ward off dementia. It does but there are benefits beyond that. The very act of trying to learn, whether you do or not, gets you out and amongst other people. That social connectivity has benefits. Making friends has health benefits we'll talk about in the 'Hang' section. Extending your social network could connect you to people from which comes new customers or business partners or spouses, all of which could lead you to a longer, healthier and happier life. (Could...)

There are also the more simple and predictable outcomes from a philosophy of lifelong learning, as opposed to leaving school or university and considering yourself done with learning. Professional trainers use a rule of thumb called the 70/20/10 principle. 70% of learning occurs in our jobs while we are doing actual work. 20% occurs during times when we are being coached or trained on the job. 10% of learning occurs in formal and scheduled classroom-type sessions. Personally, I learned how to change the battery on my keyring garage door remote control recently. I learned it via a YouTube video. I learned the opening bars to Pink Floyd's 'Wish You Were Here' the same way. I don't think I'll ever be a great or professional musician but I feel alive and alert whenever I walk away from those learning situations.

A bit more money might mean you don't delay going to a Doctor and they catch that thing you didn't know you had before it's too late. A bit more learning does equate to a bit more money but not that much really. A degree if you get it early in life does average out at lifelong earnings that are 10% higher. Bear in mind, the poets will be dragging down that average from the engineers and lawyers.

Workplace learners do earn more. Maybe that is the impact of the learning but research also suggest it might be that managers select people to receive the learning that they believe have potential. It is more that belief held by the managers that results in promotions and wage increases than the learning. I say, that if you decline the learning opportunities, the manager's belief in you will evaporate quickly.

So, evidence of learning is not necessarily a ticket to a lifestyle paved with gold but it does significantly increase your chances of getting a job at all. The longitudinal study by Dorsett, Liu and Weale concluded in 2010 showed that when you look at wages and employability together over the long term, it does pay to get your evidence of learning up.

A 2010 study by Cooper et al found that lifelong learners had:

- A more positive outlook on their future,
- A greater sense of control over their lives,
- Better health,
- Higher levels of social and civic engagement,
- Greater resilience in the face of external crises.

Leon Feinstein from The Centre for Research on the Wider Benefits of Learning in London published a study in 2012 on the effects on depression and obesity of learning efforts. Going from zero qualifications to a level 1 qualification lessens the odds of depression by 10%. For people with zero qualifications, gaining a level 1 qualification lowered your odds of obesity by 5-7%.

Beyond better jobs, higher wages and using that money to eat better and pay for Doctors, living the attitude that learning is a lifelong need puts you in situations that generate other longevity and health benefits we'll cover in more detail in other sections:

- By developing as-yet-unfulfilled potential you remove one potential source of frustration, regret and stress which cause inflammation and illness,

- You become more resilient to the stresses of change. By being proactive you take control of that change and get used to it, perhaps in a small way at first. People do not resist change; People resist being changed.

- You retain a self-perception of being an active contributor to society. As you age and re-enrol in classes, the comments you make in tutorials are useful to others as well. That sense of involvement and contribution keeps you alive longer and better,

- In signing up for classes or joining online forums on specialist topics of interest, you meet new people. Some may become new friends or other relationships.

When it comes to memory, avoid distractions as inattention is a primary cause of forgetting. Absentmindedness is often associated with getting older. We walk into a room and stand blankly wondering why we did. Leaving the mall, you may forget where you parked your car but that is primarily a factor of not having paid enough attention at the time you parked it, not necessarily some terrible cerebral degeneration. The basic skill of successful remembering, at whatever age, is to focus and concentrate on the present moment.

Not long after I first read Buettner's book "Blue Zones', I ran a 10-day programme in conjunction with a power company, local Maori and the Ministry of Social Development. The power company had a call centre with high staff turnover and a need to fill quarterly hiring intakes. The Iwi had a lot of members who were long-term unemployed and a possibility that they might invest tribal funds into the power company in the near future. And the Ministry had some quotas to get people off the unemployment benefit and into work.

So, I ran my programme which was part call centre skills, part job-seeker skills and part leadership development, team-building and problem solving. It was a bit like the TV show survivor but in reverse because if people dropped out of the programme before the end, it meant that they'd gotten a job. We lost five that way. Most pleasing for me.

This is why I put 'Teach' in parentheses after 'Learn' in the heading of this section. Developing that programme and dealing with those people provoked a lot in me and I was on my toes the entire time. They presented me with a flax kete and a carved bone necklace afterwards. Quite touching. Many of us still stay in touch, thanks to FaceBook.

During the programme, they all progressed at very different paces so I was often plugging people into tasks and sometimes having to come up with extra-for-experts on the fly. I got them to complete the online Blue Zones life expectancy app. The New Zealand average life expectancy is around 80 and mine ranged from 89 to 99, depending on if I followed their advice. One woman came up with a number of 64. I was a bit rattled and wondered if I should have thought this through a bit more before slapping people in the face with that kind of news. I paused for a few moments as I pondered my response. Before I could respond, she piped up that she was "stoked," as no one in her family had made it as far as 64 before.

Maori in New Zealand do not fare well in the life expectancy stakes and much of this can be attributed to the historical baggage and consequences of colonisation. Yet individuals can thrive and for many, their circumstances can change. It's a massive challenge to society and Governments and Maori collectives themselves to do something for large groups of people. I doubt I can help large groups of anyone. I think I helped 20. I know I can help one – one at a time. That's why I write books and why I lead training programmes.

Teaching can be the most powerful form of learning and those 10 days certainly were for me.

5.3.2.3

Challenge

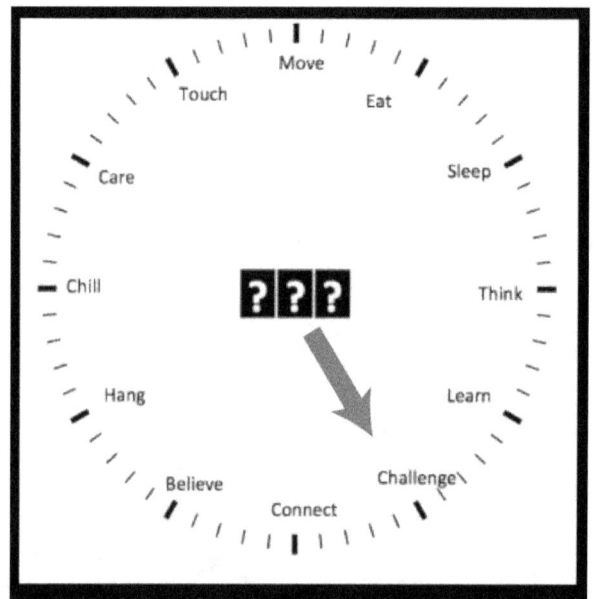

Being needed keeps you alive longer,

Avoid suffering regret by taking on challenges,

There is a simple, easy process to build new positive habits.

"I never get bored." – Jeanne Calment
(1875-1997)

Multiple studies have shown that the vast majority of regrets people have nearing the end of their lives is not what they did, but what they didn't do. They regretted inactions, not actions.

Responsibility and being needed aren't just things that society tries to convince us we *should* have because it's morally virtuous. They're things that keep us alive, purposefully active and connected. Another Ellen Langer study, this time with Judith Rodin, was on nursing home residents. They created two groups. One group were encouraged to make decisions for themselves – where and when to receive visitors for example. They were given a houseplant to look after. The other group were equally as looked after but were not offered the responsibilities. They were given the houseplants but told not to worry about them and that they would be looked after for them.

The mortality rate of the group with added purpose was half that of the other group.

Your body and mind gets used to a constant amount and grade of workload. You do not build muscle by lifting the same weight over and over again. The entire basis of progressive resistance training is that, as your body does get used to workload, you increase the workload. The body adapts. Our physiology is set up for this.

In the year 2000, my kids were 2 and 4. I was 32 and in a bit of a rut. Sameness and routine enveloped me. One day as I observed my children getting excited that the sky was blue once more, something I had long ago gotten desensitised too, I decided that I would like to recapture that sense of childlike appreciation and discovery for myself. And so I began something that I now refer to as 'My thing.' My thing is doing two new dangerous things a year. You may have new year's resolutions. I have only one and it's always the same every year – to do two new dangerous things. Although the two things do vary. That's the point.

That first year my two things were snow skiing and performing stand-up comedy. That's how I got into being a stand-up comedian and how I learned not to go snow skiing again. Over the years since, I've night-bungeed, gotten tattoos and sung 'Wild Thing' in front of 200 people. I've quit a job. I've re-established a relationship. Well, that last one might be dangerous to me. I'll find out.

The antithesis of challenge is boredom. Thomas Goetz of the University of Konstanz and the Thurgau University of Teacher Education in Konstanz, Germany study boredom.

They've identified five types as reported by National Geographic:

1. Indifferent boredom

    *   Pleasant

    *   Zoned out

2. Callibrating boredom

    *   Daydreaming

    *   Searching for new actions

3. Searching boredom

    *   Random actions

    *   Goofing around

4. Reactant boredom

    *   Restlessness, aggression

    *   Can't leave

5. Apathetic boredom

    *   Unpleasant

    *   Associated with depression

None of the boredom styles are especially useful, although I can see an argument in favour of deliberate periods of 'zoning out.' The lower down the list, the more harmful the boredom types get – to ourselves and to others. Before we get to the lower stages, we'd be well advised to self steer into some deliberate challenges.

Nassim Taleb in his book 'Antifragile' writes about how just as human bones get stronger when subjected to stress and tension, many things in life benefit from stress, disorder, volatility, and turmoil. What Taleb has identified and calls antifragile are things that not only gain from chaos but *need* chaos in order to survive and flourish. I think, to a degree, your entire life is one of those things, as long as you get to initiate and control the chaos.

> *Rather life on a rollercoaster than a conveyor belt.*

The challenge doesn't have to be dangerous or big. If you're right-handed, spend some time attempting things with your left hand. Rearrange your kitchen cupboards so you're operating less out of habit. Tackle a foreign language.

The problem with challenges is that they're challenging. Many people try to give up unhelpful behaviours, break old habits and start new helpful behaviours. Many people give up because challenges are challenging. One psychologist promoting his programme is BJ Fogg. In our attempts to take up doing 100 push-ups a day, we fail because 100 push-ups a day is hard. He suggests trying 1 push-up a day.

Doing 1 push-up a day might have zero impact on your pectoral and tricep muscle development but it will work out some new behavioural 'muscles' – your *changing muscles*. He recommends taking lots of tiny first steps at once. Do 1 push-up. Floss 1 tooth. He argues there are only two effective ways we can change our behaviour in the long term:

1. Change our environment (physical, social, work),

2. Take baby steps.

We don't lack the skill or knowledge that we should floss all our teeth all the time. (Remember the connection between gum disease and heart disease and memory loss? You don't? Uh-oh.) We know and we know we should. What we lack is the *automaticity*. That's what the baby steps get us. They make the unfamiliar positive behaviour become habitual. Once they become habitual, automaticity kicks in and we can up the number of teeth and push-ups and whatever else you target as a result of reading this book.

Fogg argues that behaviour is a function of motivation, ability and triggers that provide a call to action for the behaviour. He represents it graphically like this:

The baby step / tiny habit point is the bullseye icon. What, asked Fogg, are these triggers and how can we use them to stimulate and nurture new positive habits. Fogg answered himself by tagging the new habits to existing ones, using 'After-Then' statements.

- **After** I brush my teeth → **Then** I will floss one tooth,

- **After** I make the bed → **Then** I will do one push-up,

- **After** I enter the house after work → **Then** I will kiss my wife.

Required parameters are missing or incorrect.

Amy Maas in stuff.co.nz writes of Associate Professor Doug Elliffe, head of the University of Auckland's School of

Psychology and a specialist in human behaviour, putting down the lure of the reward to the law of effect.

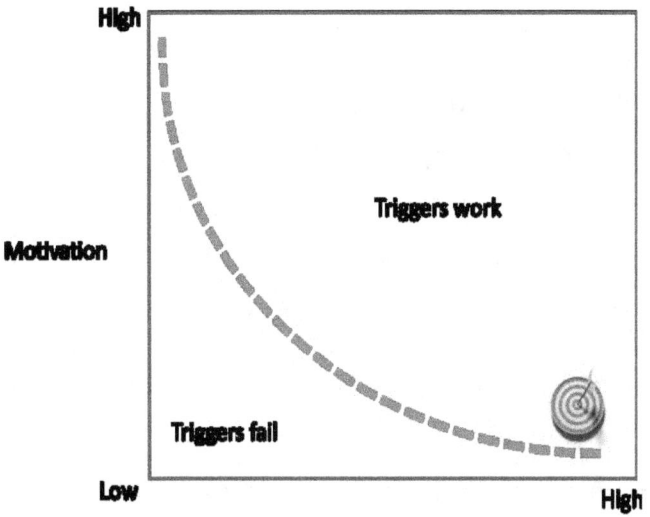

"Habit, if you like, is patterns of behaviour that are reinforced [and] therefore become repeated a lot," he says.

"When we do anything, there's probably a reinforcer maintaining that habit and then leading in some way or another into something that we want."

"Exercise programmes concentrate on that; they're trying to find ways of making it enjoyable. Reinforcers are about feeling good about yourself. It isn't about somebody coming and giving you something external. It is acting consistently with your own image of yourself."

Remember the Heath brothers and their emotional elephant with its rational rider? Their approach to behaviour change is in three parts:

Direct the rider,

- Look for bright spots / Identify those who have succeeded & how,

- Clearly & specifically script the critical moves,

131

- Point at the destination,

Motivate the elephant,

- Find the feeling,
- Shrink the change,
- Grow your people,

Shape the path,

- Tweak the environment,
- Build habits,
- Rally the herd.

2b and 3b are aligned with Fogg's process. 2c and 3c are aligned with Baumeister's and Mischel's buddy system.

Challenge your existing behaviours that aren't adding value to your life. Many of us have food rituals that we may not even be aware of. Can you go to the cinema and watch a film without popcorn or jaffas or sneaking in 400 grams of pick n mix candy from the mall supermarket? Studies from the Carlson School of management and the Harvard Business Scholl noted that participants actually perceived food as more flavoursome and enjoyable if part of a personalised and experiential ritual. This was as true for chocolate as it was for carrots. If you have a carrot-related ritual, keep it to yourself but if you're trying to cut back on the added-sugar types of chocolate, you may have to start by challenging your rituals and breaking some patterns.

My son recently joined the same social basketball team as me. I play for a men's B-grade social basketball team on a Tuesday night. Half the team are about 50 years of age and half are about 20. Half the team can jump and half the team can think. Rarely do any of us do both at the same time. I was going to quit two seasons ago but my seventeen year-old son joined the team and that's been quite the motivation for me to extend my playing days. I enjoy winning but my real sense of satisfaction comes from finishing a game in one piece.

It became quite our ritual to get takeaways on the way home from the game. My daughter is usually waiting for dinner also and often these are late nights. When our team won, I would declare how much I was looking forward to the celebration burger. When our team lost, I would admit how much I needed the commiseration burger. When my son reminded me that they were exactly the same burger, I would smirk and sigh, "No they're not. They taste very different."

That's a food ritual. I still enjoy the occasional burger but I no longer attribute icon status to grilled meat on refined white bread buns with sugar-laden condiments.

Research does provide a ring of truth to my celebration versus commiseration burger paradigm. Our perceptions of experiences are genuinely affected by what happens immediately prior to those experiences. This is called *perceptual contrast*. This is one of my favourite experiments and it's also a party trick you can try at home – or preferably, someone else's home!

Get 3 buckets. Fill one with room temperature water, one with water as cold as you can make it and the third with water as hot as you can bear. Immerse one arm in the hot bucket and the other arm in the cold bucket for a minute. Then transfer both arms into the medium bucket. It will blow your mind. Your cold arm will perceive the medium water as hot and your hot arm will perceive the medium water as cold *at the same time*. Our perceptions are highly influenced by whatever has occurred immediately beforehand.

It was the same with my ritual burgers. By creating, a binary set of possible outcomes (win or lose), both of which can be satisfied with a burger (and only satisfied with a burger), I had left myself no choice. Cunning stuff from my ravenous elephant.

If you worry about putting yourself out there with new challenges, like a bush walk or similar daunting effort or even something less daunting like reducing burger consumption, consider these research findings. <u>During</u> such arduous outings by newcomers, such as a cycle tour where it rained every day, 61% of participants reported being disappointed. <u>After</u> the activity, of those same participants, only 11% recalled being disappointed.

So, as tough as a challenge looks as we anticipate it and as we plough into it, we won't look back on it in quite the same negative light.

When it comes to challenges, the centenarians appreciate the benefits of having something to look forward to and the need to achieve completion and close loops. Their advice? Make plans for next year.

"None are so old as those who have outlived enthusiasm." – Henry David Thoreau

5.3.2.4

Connect

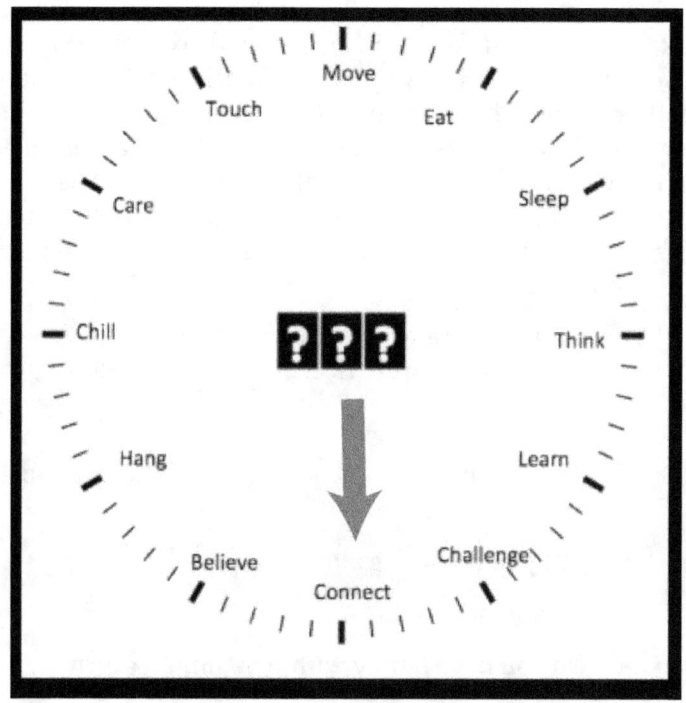

Social networks are the biggest influence on the quality and quantity of our lives,

Socialability lessens Dementia,

We need new friends & to nuture current good friends.

Social networks present an important, perhaps the most important, means of improving and protecting our positive life pathway. The groups with whom we associate determine the person we become. As we get older, we need people more than we need dollars. We need close but independent families.

Norway ranks the highest for social wellbeing. Out of 23 nations in the Sovereign Wellbeing Index, New Zealand was ranked 22nd, ahead only of Bulgaria. No disrespect to Bulgaria but ouch. Kiwis collectively score poorly on feeling lonely, meeting socially, helping out others in your local area, being treated with respect, feeling close to people in your local area, and trusting most people. These are high drivers of health and longevity and overall. Kiwis are not doing well. Only a quarter of us meet socially with friends, relatives or work colleagues more than once a week.

The more genuine and diverse connections you have, the more health benefits accrue. How many boxes below can you tick?

- Are you in a happy & healthy romantic relationship?

- Are you not living alone?

- Do you have pets?

- Do you have family within 30 minutes' drive?

- Do you have weekly family visits?

- Do you have a regular posse of friends?

- Do you have a special (call at 3am level) friend?

- Do you socialise with work people?

- Do you laugh often?

- Do you have a hobby that gets you out with others?

- Do you do any volunteer work?

A social engagement study of Japanese-American men living in Hawaii ranked the factors having the biggest association on Dementia reduction:

1. Marital status

2. Living arrangement

3. Participation in group activities

4. Participation in social events

5. A confidante relationship

The more of these factors the men had and the higher up the list the better, the less Dementia they had. The worst risk of Dementia was amongst those who had the higher factors but then lost them. Keep your eggs in multiple baskets. It's not just about having a few really solid and reliable relationships. We need to keep nurturing new ones. However, I am not suggesting that you cultivate a 'back-up wife.'

The Australian Longitudinal Study of
Aging found that people aged 70 or more
with active social lives lived 22% longer.

Even television might help us connect, despite being slammed for making us more isolated and prone to manipulation by marketers into poor food choices and meaningless and never-ending mass consumerism, all while sat motionless on a couch decaying away. Just turning a TV on and watching whatever is on is mindless and no substitute for genuine human connection. But if you do live alone or are immobile for a period, then TV and the internet can help connect you to a degree. Any positive connection is better than no connection. If you're a fan of a quality show with a good story and intellectual stimulus such as 'Breaking Bad' and you can connect to other fans via Twitter or fansites to debate the storyline, then at least that's something. If you're recording it and 'self-scheduling,' you can also lessen your exposure to adverts.

Even video games, often portrayed as the villain in the debate around the social lives of young people, can be beneficial as a driver of connection. Daniel Johnson leads the gaming research group at the Young and Well Co-operative Research Centre. He says, "Our studies of play with others have revealed benefits for young people in terms of social wellbeing and feelings of relatedness. But importantly, we have also found co-operative video game play to be associated with increased brain activity for younger people.

"More broadly, using a well-validated measure of mental health and wellbeing, we have found evidence that for adult players, a positive impact on wellbeing resulted from playing video games with other people. In a randomised controlled trial with a clinically depressed sample of adults, the positive influences of video games have been shown to include a reduction in tension, anger, depression and fatigue and increase in vigour.

"Importantly, these improvements were supported by associated changes in brain activity and heart rate variability. Research focusing on video game play among children has suggested that the best outcomes are associated with moderate video game play as opposed to no play or excessive play. These benefits have extended to greater positive emotions, having less risky friendship networks, better self-esteem and higher levels of family closeness.

Researchers at the University of Rochester, New York, have shown that whether people engage with video games in a healthy way is a consequence of whether certain basic needs (feelings of competence, autonomy and relatedness) are being met in their lives.

If your needs are not being met and you are less satisfied in your everyday life, you are more likely to engage unhealthily with video games and for play to result in less enjoyment and more tension.

In contrast, if you are broadly happy and satisfied, you are more likely to engage with video games in a balanced, healthy way and your video game playing is likely to lead to feelings of enjoyment and increased energy.

It's not enough to merely connect. You can enhance the benefits of connecting by making commitments.

5.3.3

Social

We've looked at the Physical and Mental controls for enhancing our productive life and health spans. The third leg of the trifecta is the five Social controls. A better metaphor than trifecta might be a three-legged stool. An over-emphasis on the Physical and the Mental without addressing the available Social controls leads to the whole thing falling over. In fact, the evidence might surprise you. The social aspect might be the most powerful control you have for health and life, more so than diet or exercise. And, of course, they are all interconnected.

It all rests on a fundamental question. <u>Why</u> would anyone want to live longer and be more productive? The answer to that question is almost certain to have social meaning. We want it for partners, families, friends, our home town or who ever. The answer to the *why* is almost always a *who*...

5.3.3.1

Believe

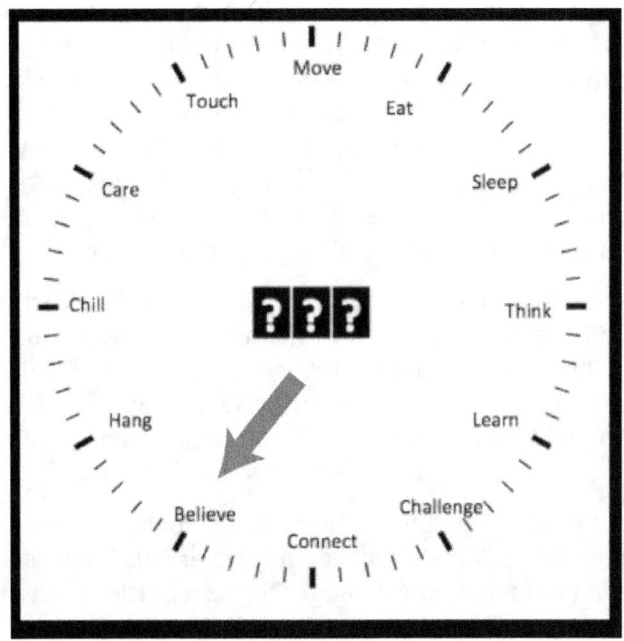

There needs to be a point,

Our perceptions affect our responses,

Beliefs affects physiology, even the efficacy of meds.

Religion's job was to keep us quiet and in line with the status quo and to prepare us for death.

Richard Dawkins asks, "If you take religion away, what are you going to put in its place? What have you to offer the dying patients, the weeping bereaved, the lonely Eleanor Rigbys for whom God is their only friend?" My thought would be a hug.

Us non-believers might get all self righteous at how religious people are deluded but they get benefits beyond our feelings of smug self-righteousness. People attending at least one religious service a week reduce their mortality rate by twenty percent. Those of us who never attend any have a fifty percent increase. Of those who never attend, their rate of mortality due to infectious disease, respiratory disease or diabetes is 400% higher. People with an active religious involvement are experiencing lives 29% longer. Perhaps these people derive benefits from behaviours of gratitude and acceptance, optimism (optimists live 23% longer), coping skills and, perhaps most important of all, it gives life a point.

Believing isn't all about faith or belief in God or Doctor Who. It is about values. I do believe in values. Not necessarily your values but I am sure that values exist. Maybe we'd like to change ours or those of the people we lead or love? The key is to get a foot in the door – some little commitments towards the shift.

How else do our beliefs impact our health and productive lifespan? Brian Wansick ran a study where his team relabelled bottles of red wine they'd bought for $2 a bottle, locally known as 'Two Buck Chuck.' All were relabelled similarly as Noah's Winery but there were two subtle variations. Half were noted as being a product of California and half a product of North Dakota. The research team presumed people would be more favourably disposed towards the wines labelled as being from a traditional wine producing area and be averse to the wine supposedly from a region unknown for wine production. No doubt there were other preconceptions about California versus North Dakota.

All diners were given a free glass of wine – half got 'California' and half got 'North Dakota.' Both groups drank the same amount of wine but the North Dakota group rated the

142

food they got served much lower, despite it being the same food everyone got. The California group stayed 20% longer and ate 11% more food. In debriefings, 99% of diners denied the possibility that they could have been influenced by the wine's labelling.

In 2009, Barbara Muller at Radboud University in Nijmegen ran a study with smokers aged 17 to 47. One group were asked to read out loud a prepared list of anti-smoking arguments that they'd been given. The other group were asked to come up with a list of anti-smoking arguments by themselves and write it down. Both then encountered a convenient and fake thirty minute delay, thanks to the researchers.

In the downtime, 36.8% of the smokers who had read the prepared list of anti-smoking arguments did not light up. What percentage refrained from smoking amongst the group that had come up with their own anti-smoking arguments? 70.6%. This is the power of a small commitment of emotional investment. Instead of telling a teenage child of yours or an employee that they need to be more organised, you'll get better results if you ask them, "If you were more organised, what might some benefits be?"

Belief has physical effects. Cancer patients whose course of treatment includes chemotherapy are given written and verbal explanations of the process, potential benefits, risks and side effects and then the treatment commences. Many of those people experience the predicted side effects _before_ the treatment commences.

You've probably heard of the 'Placebo Effect' where drug trials include a proportion of recipients who receive a pill that is not actually the medicine being tested but a substitute sugar pill. Often, patients report benefits even though they received a Placebo. The opposite is the 'Nocebo Effect.' This is a common problem in pharmaceutical trials. A 1980s study found that heart patients were far more likely to suffer side-effects from their blood-thinning medication if they had first been warned of the medication's side-effects.

But let's get back to the concept of 'Believe' in a spiritual sense. You might believe in God or another God or a range of Gods, Doctor Who, or none of the above. Gods came about from our primitive tribal times to help us explain what to us then was utterly unexplainable and pretty soon after to act as a control system for those with power over the masses. Accept your crappy time in this life and you'll rock it out in the next one – just don't kill the King.

These days, it's all nonsense right? Well, not exactly. God or no God, there are benefits to having beliefs and especially if you share them with others and most of all if there are some lifestyle constraining rules in this belief system that do actually help us out physically, socially and psychologically. For example, a Sabbath or alternative day of rest is a really good idea. Not because God will feel disrespected without one but because it's a good idea to have a break. It's even better to spend that break with some people who like you and with whom you feel a sense of belonging, engaged in some positive, affirming rituals. A lot of religions will give you some of that.

Regardless of the facts of the existence of any God or Gods, here are some benefits for 'Believers':

- Higher self-esteem,
- Adapt better to bereavement,
- Feel less lonely,
- Less likely to suffer from Depression,
- Make faster recovery from Depression,
- Less likely to commit suicide,
- Less likely to suffer anxiety,

- Display fewer psychotic tendencies (other than believing in an invisible friend of course),

- Lower likelihood of youth delinquency and criminal activity,

- Greater marital stability,

There was even one study showing that Christian teenagers were 90% less likely to contract meningococcal disease. I guess they do as they they're told and they're told not to share spit.

There are an increasing number of, for want of a better word, 'movements' around the world to pick out the good bits and strip away all the irrelevant or harmful historical baggage and control structures. One such is 'The Sunday Assembly.' They currently number only a few thousand people but are spreading around the world. Their slogan is, "A global network of super people who want to make the most out of this one life we know we have." They claim their assemblies with speeches and songs will energise, vitalise, restore, repair, refresh and recharge. "No matter what the subject of the Assembly, it will solace worries, provoke kindness and inject a touch of transcendence into the everyday." I'm not a member nor am I promoting them especially. It does strike me though that what they are focusing on are what I called 'The Good Bits.'

At some point, they'll probably start collecting money. This leads to many of 'The Bad Bits.'

5.3.3.2

Hang

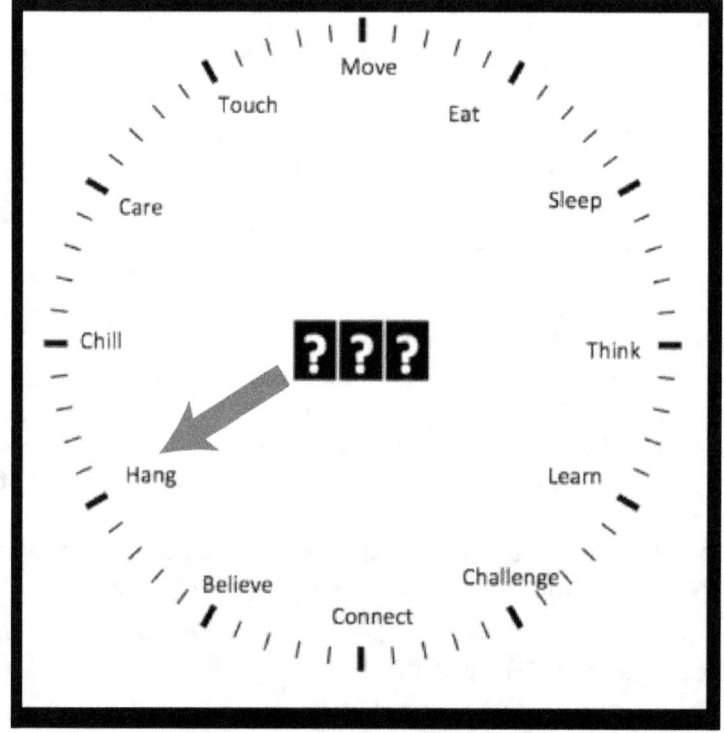

The health benefits of friendships fade without effort
to maintain them,

People with social support have fewer cardiovascular
problems,

Loneliness leads to higher blood pressure, anxiety
levels and poorer sleep quality.

Loneliness is a disease. Conversely, hanging with true friends can cure or, at least, prevent or mitigate actual diseases. Socialability is a double edged sword – it depends who you socialise with. <u>Good</u> friends are good for you but not all friends are good friends.

A study published in the journal *Cancer* followed women with Ovarian cancer. Those with high levels of social support had lower levels in their blood of a protein called Interleukin 6 (IL-6.) This protein is linked to cancer aggression. This group also responded better to treatment. Those with low levels of social support had 70% higher levels of IL-6 and in the organ where the tumour was, the levels were 250% higher.

A study by David Siegel published in *Lancet* found in women with breast cancer that high levels of social support doubled the survival and recovery odds, as well as lowering reported levels of pain.

This isn't all touchy-feely stuff. There are simple practical benefits in having a close network of friends. Quite apart from the emotional support, for which there are demonstrable physiological positives, they can provide resources and information as well as advocate for you when you may well be least able to. They can round up others or raise money or do things for you. This is obvious and simple, yet dangerously impactful when absent. Maybe your butler could do a lot of that if you had a butler? You'd probably need a team of butlers. This might be the screenplay to the movie *Arthur 3*. (Here, good friends would tell you that there should never be an *Arthur 3*. There should never have been a second one.)

Tom Valeo on WebMD.com wrote: "People with social support have fewer cardiovascular problems and immune problems, and lower levels of cortisol -- a stress hormone," says Tasha R. Howe, PhD, associate professor of psychology at Humboldt State University. "Why? The evolutionary argument maintains that humans are social animals, and we have evolved to be in groups. We have always needed others for our survival.

It's in our genes. Therefore, people with social connections feel more relaxed and at peace, which is related to better health."

"One thing research shows is that as one's social network gets smaller, one's risk for mortality increases. And it's a strong correlation - almost as strong as the correlation between smoking and mortality."

Lonely young people participate disproportionately in illicit drug use. They have higher blood pressure, anxiety levels and poorer sleep quality. (Even the ones not on illicit drugs.) And Americans, at least, are getting lonelier. A study in the *American Sociological Review* looking at 1985-2004 found a 33% reduction in people who a friend with whom they could discuss serious life issues. The ratio of people who only had family members with whom they could discuss serious life issues rose from 57% to 80%. The ratio of people who only had a spouse with whom to discuss serious life issues went from 5% to 9%. This is tough when the serious life issue you need to discuss is your spouse.

Denmark's doing OK though. Sociologists suppose the colder weather of the Scandinavian countries keep people indoors and in groups more often so social norms have developed over the centuries to reinforce this. FaceBook and smartphones can only destroy this to a degree. Certainly they're happier and more social than the average American.

Lonely people, especially men, are more prone to accidents, suicide, heart disease, anxiety and depression. A Swedish study found that having no close friends increased the risk of a first-time heart attack by 50%. Women with close friends have lower blood pressure, less frequency of diabetes and are less likely to have excess abdominal fat. Social ties lessen the body's damaging internal inflammation.

People describing or remembering stressful situations have lower blood pressure when they have a supportive friend by their side. People are more likely to eat fruit and vegetables, exercise regularly and quit smoking if they have an effective and positive network of friends and family.

Friendship does work both ways. The act of helping out a friend has similar positive effects on your physiology. Having a happy friend who lives within a mile of you increases your own chances of personal happiness by 25%. But the downsides work both ways too. Having an overweight friend increases your own chances of becoming overweight by 57%.

There is also the negative impact of what psychologists call 'co-ruminating.' Ruminating is when cows re-chew over the contents of their multiple stomachs. Ruminating is a psychological metaphor for thinking about negative stuff over and over again, compelling your body to re-experience al the stress and unhappiness hormones all over again. The body can't tell the difference between an actual and current experience, and one you're ruminating over, so you get to stew in your own juices for much longer. 'Co-Ruminating' is when a friend does it to you about their negative experiences and your body starts boosting stress hormone production on their behalf in sympathy. By all means, be a mate and hear out friends with a beef but a good friend will tell them when to put a plug in it for both your sakes. Go for a walk and flush those hormones out of your system. Or listen to some upbeat music. Or go find that elusive third good friend.

Putting your money and discretionary time towards shared experiences has been shown to optimise our happiness. Material possessions become part of the background; Experiences get better with time. Especially when the following conditions are met:

- Brings you together with other people, fostering a sense of social connection,

- Makes a memorable story that you can enjoy retelling (or embellishing) for years to come,

149

- Strongly linked to the sense of who you are or who you wish to be,

- A unique or incomparable opportunity.

Quite apart from the emotion-health connection, having friends and loved ones means that there is someone else besides yourself reminding you to take your pills, calling an ambulance or advocating for you in hospital. That's all good for upping your odds when times get tough.

Social norming affects our behaviour and choices. Jeni Cross studied anti-litter campaigns in Colorado. One campaign used photos and displays showing how much litter got dropped on streets each day. The theory was that seeing how much litter people dropped would shame citizens into using bins. What actually happened is that they made people believe that most people littered and that social norming actually drove an increase in littering behaviour.

Hotels are keen for the environment's sake and for the sake of lowering their own expenses for their guests to re-use their towels and decrease laundry volumes. The most effective method is informing guests the percentage of other guests who re-use their towels. The last hotel I stayed at the number was 42%. That's probably enough to drive social norming and greater re-use. I wonder now if 42% was a true figure?

Gossip isn't just morally reprehensible, it is also a terrible socialisation strategy. John Skowronski of Ohio University studied trait transference. People assign to the gossiper the negative traits of others that they are gossiping about.

But the sharing of news amongst friends is a powerful social reinforcer and the age-old premise of a 'Happy Hour' seems to provide a useful ritual, as long as you keep to no more than two drinks and stand up.

5.3.3.3

Chill

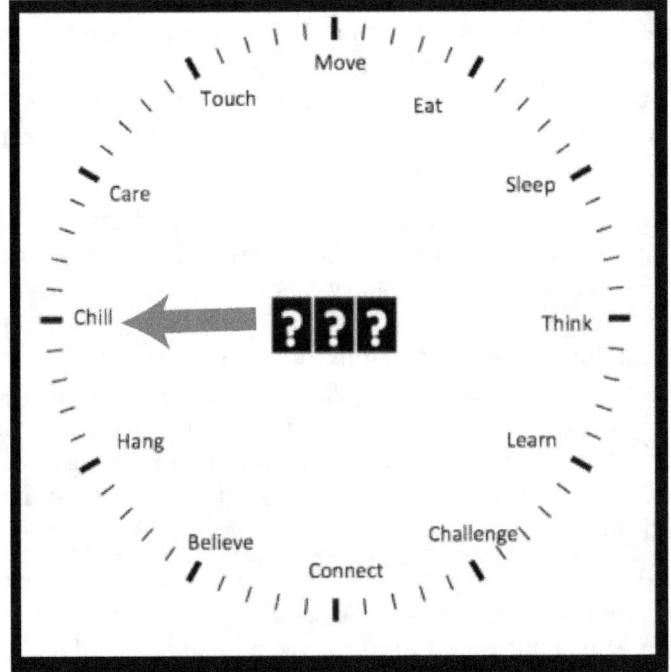

Tension contributes to internal inflammation – a major health problem,

Over time, stress hormones damage you,

Perpetual 'busyness' is damaging the relationships your later survival will rely on.

Live, Work, Love

Our cells and ourselves as a whole can be in a catabolic state or an anabolic state. Both are essential for our survival. Basically, anabolic is a building state and catabolic is a cleaning-up state. This makes sense to me. A bit of work needs to be followed by a bit of rest and a clean-up, whether that's us at the gym or the office or it's the cells in our liver after a party at the office. Our busy modern western lives and diets make us disproportionately anabolic.

A very basic species-level analysis would find that we are dumb and sexy when anabolic but smart and hungry when catabolic. From an evolutionary perspective, our caveman world was at any one time either full of food or scarce of food. Our physiology adapted to cope. In the good times, we got anabolic and got laid. In the lean times, we got catabolic and got smart so we could find food as soon as possible and hopefully get laid later. I don't think I'm over-simplifying things here. Even in modern times, when we go on a third date, dinner comes first.

In 2004, Nobel Prize winner Elizabeth Blackburn proved that chronic stress over time accelerates cellular aging. She said that some form of meditation may have salutary effects on Telomere length. (Remember – that's our inbuilt cellular life-timer.)

People are like rubber bands. Stretch them too much and they snap, damaged, perhaps irreparably so. Never stretch them at all and they just lie there useless, without purpose, the world unaware of and unaffected by their existence. But stretch them, a little at first, then increasingly more-so, and they'll serve a valuable purpose.

The physiological stress response from our caveman days caused by our brain's survival surge in flight or flight situations releases many hormones into our system as our body seeks to engage or avoid a perceived threat. Gone are sabre toothed tigers but the instinct remains and we react in the same crude fashion to modern threats, real or imagined. One is cortisol which is great for thickening blood if we're about to get beaten up and anticipating needing to heal in a hurry. But if we're just stressed by motorway traffic, a jerk of a boss or a disobedient teenager then that same cortisol will boost your blood pressure, boost your blood sugar and suppress your immunity. Sabre toothed tiger fights were rare but motorway traffic, jerk bosses and disobedient teenagers are constant. That cortisol, over time, will kill you.

A Swedish study of 3000 workers found that those who perceived their bosses to be incompetent were 24% more likely to end up with a serious heart health issue. Conversely a Gallup study of people aged over 95 found that the average age of 'retirement' was 80 and that they had always considered their work to be 'fun.'

> *"If we do not change our direction, we are likely to end up where we are headed." –*
> *Ancient proverb. (Let's say it was Chinese to give it a bit more mystique.)*

Perhaps easier said than done, but if you felt that life was too busy, it isn't going to change itself. Various studies offered some advice:

- Find an hour a day to play,
- Cure yourself of 'the disease to please',
- Create a 'zone of your own',
- Book 'restoration days',
- Declutter

- Make plans rather than being perpetually reactive,

- Listen,

- Walk.

The damaging source of workplace stress is not the work itself but conflict with other people. You can either change your situation or change your mental response to the situation.

Check out the 'Slow Food' movement. British Doctor Malcolm Kendrick noted the obvious 400% difference in coronary heart diseases between the USA and France. Much study has gone into the 'what' of their diet. That's where the initial impetus for the reservatrol research began. Kendrick believes it is not the 'what', it's the 'how.' Eating under stress, as the typical American with heart disease does, raises insulin levels and blood sugar levels, creating the metabolic state that triggers atherosclerotic plaque development. That is a primary driver of coronary heart disease

Limit what you try to do each day. Don't confuse activity with productivity. Eat meals at a table with no TV. Savour the now.

The benefits of laughter include reducing anxiety and stress, oxygenating our blood and organs, improving circulation, releasing endorphins, lifting our mood, strengthening our immune system and the best longevity booster of all – reducing our blood pressure. Our bodies can't differentiate between real laughter and unreal. We reap the benefits regardless, even from a smile. So fake it til you make it.

American comedian and actor Patton Oswalt (the voice of the rat in the movie 'Ratatouille') summed up the immune system nicely in an interview with Conan O'Brien. The aches, sniffles, etc that we get when we're sick are our immune system at work. If we take medicine to suppress them, we're helping the virus not our immune system. It's like our bodies are the building in 'Die Hard', the virus is Hans Gruber and our immune system is John McLane. Why would we help Hans Gruber? A laugh and a useful metaphor.

Western adults laugh, on average, seventeen times a day. Children average 300-400 times a day. When my daughter was younger and got a bit silly, I'd sometimes remark, "Grow up!" Her response without exception to me was, "You grow down!" I think now she surely had a good point.

Laughter and happiness aren't necessarily synonymous but they seem to be equally popular topics amongst researchers. Sonya Lyubomirsky is the most often cited happiness researcher and much of her work shows that happiness in itself has benefits but also makes for better relationships, which brings all those other physical and mental benefits we've already covered. Happiness-specific benefits include:

- Greater socialability,
- Greater altruism,
- Increases how much you like yourself and others,
- Improves ability to resolve conflict,
- Strengthens immune system
- What determines our ability to be happy?
- Self Control 40%
- Intentional Activities 10%
- Genetics 50%

Lyubomirsky found that after circumstantial changes, good or bad, our happiness will revert to its default set point but after our own intentional activities, it maintains its higher levels for longer. She has an iPhone app called 'Live Happy' that might be worth a micro investment. Her suggestions for intentional activities that can drive up your happiness include exercises in practicing optimism when imagining the future, savouring life's pleasures in the here and now, and the importance of staying active. She found that performing five non-financial acts of kindness per day raised people's happiness by 40%. It can't be too hard to hold the door open for someone five times a day. (Just make sure, it's not a pull door before you push it; Otherwise your act of kindness will be making the person behind you giggle.)

One thing that prevents many of us from chilling is making decisions and one thing that has been proven to make decision-making more difficult, more stressful and less effective is having too many choices. Having too many choices can be mentally paralysing. The New York Times wrote of the famous 'Jam' Study:

Sheena Iyengar, a professor of business at Columbia University and the author of "The Art of Choosing," conducted the study in 1995.

In a California gourmet market, Professor Iyengar and her research assistants set up a booth of samples of jams. Every few hours, they switched from offering a selection of 24 jams to a group of six jams. On average, customers tasted two jams, regardless of the size of the assortment, and each one received a coupon good for $1 off one jam.

Here's the interesting part. Sixty percent of customers were drawn to the large assortment, while only 40 percent stopped by the small one. But 30 percent of the people who had sampled from the small assortment decided to buy jam, while only 3 percent of those confronted with the two dozen jams purchased a jar.

That study "raised the hypothesis that the presence of choice might be appealing as a theory," Professor Iyengar said, "but in reality, people might find more and more choice to actually be debilitating."

This has been shown to not only apply to jam but to financial planning and dating. "Yeah, I can see myself marrying him but is he 'the one'?" There is no *one*. Make your choice and live with it. The alternative is growing old alone sharing jam with your cats. So says, Lori Gottlieb, the author of 'Marry Him: The Case for Settling for Mr. Good Enough.' (The cat and jam remark was mine, not hers.)

Regardless of any Gods or wizards you might believe in, one of the upsides for health and state of mind routinised by some religions is the concept of a Sabbath – a strictly observed day of rest. If properly observed, it's a great means of steadying the mind, plugging into family and lowering your body's internal levels of inflammation.

When you are chilling, you become more aware of the signals your own body is sending you as you can listen without the clutter and the noise. The expression 'gut feeling' doesn't just relate to notions of sixth sense or intuition, there is a truth to it. You do not want to know how the scientists Bayliss and Starling discovered this a century ago but our gut has its own nervous system. Our stomach and intestines propel food in one direction. This system of muscular contractions still functions even when all input from the brain or spine has been eliminated. Your gut has a local nervous system – a *mind of its own*. Ever been nervous? Where in your body did you feel that nervousness first? That's a gut feeling.

5.3.3.4

Care

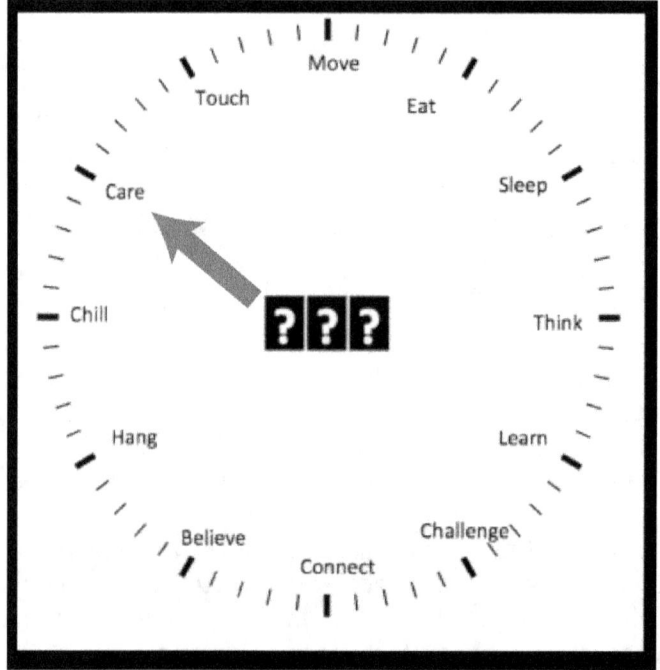

Men repressing emotions are damaging themselves *physically*,

There are practical alternatives to talking about feelings,

Apreciating the small things you have makes you healthier.

Are we becoming less caring? A survey of Christmas wishes resulted in the following:

- 2010 Peace and happiness
- 2011 iPad

That doesn't necessarily prove anything. I included it for a laugh. But if we were more interested in iPads than peace and happiness, would it matter? I don't mean would it matter in a moral sense but in a literal sense. Does caring more improve our longevity, health and enable us to be more productive? If it does, does it matter *what* we care about?

New Zealand's Mental Health Foundation promotes their five winning ways to wellbeing:

1. Talk and listen. Be there. Feel connected,

2. Give your time, your words, your presence,

3. Take notice. Remember the simple things that give you joy,

4. Keep learning. Embrace new experiences. See opportunities. Surprise yourself,

5. Be active. Do what you can. Enjoy what you do. Move your mood.

We flourish when we are being relied on. There is a necessity to being necessary.

Dr Laura Carstensen of Stanford University observed that once someone begins to consciously anticipate death, they tend to disengage – to *not care*.

It's not enough to care; you need to express that you do. Many of the books and studies I looked at emphasised how men are the ones who die first. Often, a reason cited beyond the physical ones is a general reluctance amongst men to speak freely and express emotionally. I'm not advocating a total hugfest here but men need to pick up the pace. Michelle Duff on stuff.co.nz wrote that a New Zealand Ministry of Health report shows death rates are as low as they have even been since mortality data was collected, but men are far more likely to die of preventable causes than women. Heart Foundation medical director Professor Norman Sharpe said it is a gap that will continue to widen as a "new wave" of health problems caused by obesity start showing up in the statistics. Men are up to twice as likely to die from preventable illnesses like heart disease and diabetes. In 2010, the male rate of death from coronary heart disease was 85.3 percent higher than the female rate. When it comes to dying in motor vehicle crashes and suicide, the gender gap becomes a chasm. Men are three times as likely to die in a car crash and more than twice as likely to kill themselves.

There are lots of reasons why men traditionally do not take care of themselves and do not express themselves. More important is the question of what it will take to encourage them to do so as soon as possible. Recent years have seen social media and advertising campaigns such as Movember and Blue October have highlighted mens' health issues. Celebrities have been drafted in to raise awareness. Former All Black great John Kirwan's work around depression and his book 'All Blacks Don't Cry' is an obvious and effective example of this.

Ultimately society can chip away at big changes like this. I'm more interested in what individuals like you can do right now. You need to have a powerful reason to want to change your unhelpful and unhealthy behaviours. Again, the question of why you should is probably going to be answered with a *who*. Post their picture on your car's dashboard. Next time you're on autopilot and your car is steering itself towards a fastfood drive-through, hopefully that person's image can remind you to steer away. We need powerful immediate and personal motivators to overcome ingrained behaviours, many of which have been with us since childhood.

The problem with caring about things is that you get upset when the things you care about die, leave or don't care back.

That is a risk but the research clearly shows that life as an emotional roller coaster is more worth living than a flat emotional conveyor belt.

If the Government is serious about reversing the obesity epidemic, it must introduce tough new rules on the packaging of children's treats, Consumer NZ says.

The consumer advocacy group is calling for the control of marketing gimmicks on food packaging – particularly cartoon characters, free toys and on-packet puzzles targeting children. As reported by stuff.co.nz, Consumer chief executive Sue Chetwin said under-13s were particularly susceptible to tricks of the advertising trade. With a person's lifelong food preferences formed at an early age, if companies rope them in young, they'll likely be hooked for life, the watchdog's report says.

American researchers have found children preferred the taste of McDonald's-branded food over that in plain packaging, even though both were identical – and the same effect was seen with cartoon characters like Dora the Explorer. Chetwin said licensing kids' characters from companies like Disney was costly, and companies would not invest the cash unless they knew it would pay off.

Counselling has its place but for situations that are less needing of expensive external professional intervention, try 'Expressive Writing.'

Talking about stuff is random and disorganised. The process of writing requires you to think about what's happened, its consequences, the alternatives and the future. Thinking then writing puts it into a structure and gives it meaning. And that's what our brains require – to make meaning. We see shapes in the clouds because our brains like to find meaning in randomness. Until we get meaning, we do not get closure. The Expressive Writing technique has been shown to provide a:

- Boost in a sense of personal well-being,

- Reduction in health problems,

- Increase in self-esteem and happiness.

Expressive Writing has been shown by Robert Emmons and Michael McCullough to make people happier, more optimistic, healthier and even got them exercising more. And it's not just for getting closure on traumatic events. It is equally effective for reminding us of the positive things in our lives for which we should be grateful and a gratitude attitude has physiological health benefits too. In the same way that we can walk into a room with fresh bread baking, get wowed by the smell then not notice it after a few minutes, we get desensitised. If you walk out of the room, then back in again, you re-notice the smell. Expressive Writing enables us to re-notice the positives. Once a week, make some entries in a gratitude journal. You should probably do it daily but let's start with tiny habits... Complete the following:

Weekly, when I

_____

Then I will update my gratitude journal.

A practical manifestation of caring is washing your hands. It is nothing but a hassle in the now but it saves lives. People might die from an infection caught off your dirty hands but it is unlikely. It is probable that they'll get sick. Every instance of preventable sickness is another unnecessary experience of inflammation, non homeostatis and disruption that our bodies have to endure. If we cared for ourselves and others, we'd wash our hands, as evidenced by the interior of my friend Mike's toilet door:

A survey of people declared that 91% of people washed their hands after visiting restaurant toilets. The actual truth was 82% which is less bad than I was expecting. It just means next time you and four friends are out to eat, you have to work out who that 18% of non washers at your table are. A 1992 study by the New England Journal of Medicine found that 30-48% of staff at *Intensive Care Units* did not wash their hands properly. At this point, I'll just finish by noting that Louis Pasteur refused to shake hands with anyone ever. Smart guy.

5.3.3.5

Touch

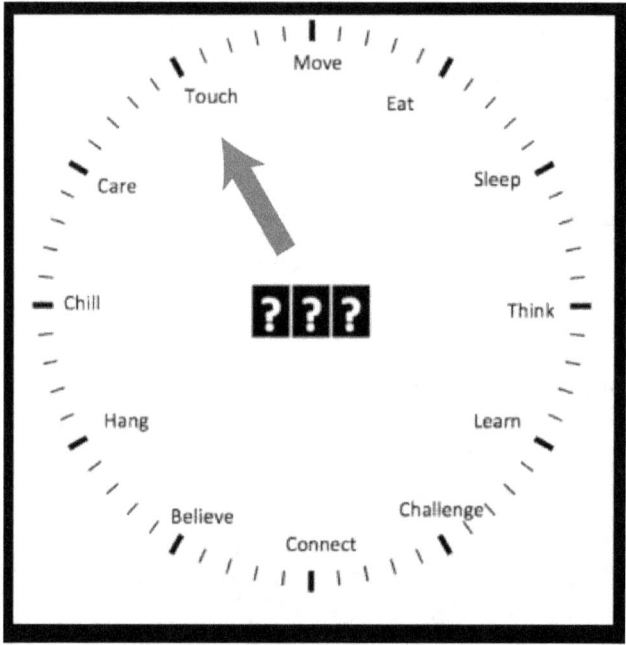

Touch stimulates oxytocin production in our bodies,

- High-touch families enjoy better health,
- High-touch teams win more,
- High-touch relationships experience more trust, honesty & helpfulness.

A study at the University of California San Diego School of Medicine found physiological benefits in skin-to-skin contact and intimate eye contact. It stimulated the release of oxytocin.

It's sometimes referred to as 'the love molecule' or the 'trust hormone.' Poets, pop singers and scientists can argue whether love is real or just a product of oxytocin exposure and over-association with another individual. Here are some benefits of naturally occurring oxytocin:

- It's easy to get via a hug or a glance,
- It's a built-in love potion,
- Enhances orgasms,
- It reinforces mother-child bonding,
- It reduces social fear,
- Healing and pain relief
- Moderates weight, reduces glucose intolerance, reduces insulin resistance,
- Antidepressant,
- Relieves stress,
- Decreases intestinal inflammation,
- Primes generosity.

I'm loathe to have my book tarred as a touchy-feely piece of pop psychology, although I'm quite keen on the "pop" bit. I haven't been an especially huggy or touchy person myself in my life so far. My research clearly shows I'm missing out on some tangible benefits that even cold, clinical all-business types would have to acknowledge.

Lewis Mehl-Madrona, Program director at the Center for Health and Healing at Beth Israel Medical Centre in New York, reported on the effects of massage. There is lessening of the activity of the hypothalamic area of the brain, which controls the fight or flight stress response. The body's level of stress hormones decreases and the level of endorphins increases, leading to a lower perception of pain and increased sense of well-being. It's not just touchy-feely mumbo-jumbo, its chemistry – brain chemistry.

In 1977, Chris Kleinke ran a study on the effects on honesty of gaze and touch. Subjects were far more likely to return money 'accidentally' left behind if they had been touched with eye contact during a brief interaction. Touch encourages honesty and who couldn't use more of that in our personal and business relationships?

April Crusco and Christopher Wetzel in 1984 ran a study on waiting staff, touching and tipping. That's an objective and tangible measure if ever there was one. One slight touch on an upper arm routinely led to bigger tips. I mentioned this study in a training course I was leading once. One woman mentioned how offended she would be by something like that. The research shows most people don't even consciously notice the touch but it is a normal distribution and the minority at the non-touchy end of the spectrum will shudder and be repelled. But the tip jar is the final arbiter and, overall, it's a wise strategy. This personal variation in comfort levels with physical contact is called Proxemics and it is learned behaviour.

Nicolas Gruguen in 2003 showed other positive impacts on behaviour of touch. After a brief interaction involving one simple touch, subjects helped the researcher pick up 'accidentally' dropped items 90% of the time, compared with 63% when no touch occurred. Helen Hamm and Frank Willis conducted a study in 1980 involving asking passers-by to sign a petition. In two versions, touch raised the signing rate from 55% to 81% and from 40% to 70%.

Who doesn't like a massage? It's obviously and inherently relaxing, right? It has other benefits too. Field's study in 1996 showed it helped subjects improve their results in maths tests. As well as higher test scores, the subjects had lower blood pressure and less of the stress hormone cortisol.

High-five anyone? Don't leave me hanging. In case you think this activity is a waste of time, think again. The touches are not just symbolic indications of encouragement, celebration and mutual support, they have actual physical consequences that contribute to results. Michael Kraus and his team studied the NBA's professional basketball teams for a year and the degree and frequency of in-game touching in which they engaged – high-fives, chest-bumps, pats-on-the-back and so forth. There was a direct correlation between high-touch teams and high-success teams.

Why might this be? Kraus believes the touch has a number of subtle but accumulative effects. Touch lowers the stress hormones in the body. Otherwise, over time these would inflate the body's exposure to inflammation which leads to more injuries and slower recovery from injuries. Winning teams are usually low-injury teams. High stress situations such as close basketball games can shut down parts of players' brains as the organ gets into survival fight or flight mode saturated by stress hormones. Lessen that and you get better decisions. More decisions of a higher quality by more players lead to more wins. Oxytocin is the trust hormone. Trust-promoting touches is a foundation of a high-trust team, critical for success in a sport where no one individual can win it all for them every time, no matter how super the super star. The study reckoned that they corrected for the possibility that it was the winning that lead to the touching and not the other way around.

For the record, that season the touchiest player (in a good sense) was Kevin Garnett.

Of course, it's not just pro team athletes but romantic couples where touch is impactful and often telling. Studies show that for the most part the couples that report the highest levels of satisfaction with their relationship are high-touch couples. Interestingly, the most critical factor is not the frequency of touching as much as it is the nature of *the response* to the initial touch.

Handshakes are a tremendous driver of social connectivity and we all have our own opinions on what constitutes an acceptable handshake and how we feel about unacceptable ones.

Handshakes are usually all business so let's segue now into our section on 'Work' and how the 12 controls, a longer and healthier life affects, and is affected by, our world at work.

WORK

> *"Work saves a man from three great evils: boredom, vice and need." – Voltaire (Real name: François-Marie Arouet. He changed it to a one-word non de plume, like Prince or Madonna. If he'd lived today, I think he would've tweeted a lot.)*

A very common piece of advice from centenarians is to spend less than you earn. A bank advert in New Zealand boldly claimed that money is neither good nor bad, it depends what you do with it. That may be true but it seems, from a health perspective, that debt sucks. I'm on the fence with this one because to get a freehold house, you need a mortgage. To build a business that outlasts you, initially you probably need a loan.

Happy Money, a book by Elizabeth Dunn and Michael Norton outlines numerous studies into how best we can use and trade-off our money to improve our lives. Doubling your income will at best only ever increase your happiness by nine percent. And above an annual income of $US75,000, additional income doesn't influence our daily happiness levels at all. They identify five core principles to guide us in our money-using decisions if happiness is what we're after:

- Buy experiences not things,
- Make treats a treat,

- Buy time,

- Pay now & Consume later (Anticipation se rejouir),

- Invest in others.

We're bad at saving for the future because we have a hard time imagining ourselves there. Hal Ersner-Hershfield from Northwestern University conducted a study with Stanford in 2010 on 'High Future Self Continuity'. They developed a mirror that gave subjects an avatar reflection of themselves as they would look *when they were seventy years old*. Compared to a control group, those having a conversation with their seventy year old selves set aside twice as much for retirement savings. The sooner they develop a smartphone app for that, the better.

Envision a future and design it. Diversify and invest, not just financially but in all aspects of your life. Nourish your social relationships. Work longer and save more. Anchor your development around lifelong learning.

Some say that the future of crap jobs belongs to robots but that potentially has its own pitfalls. A union boss was taking a tour of a Ford car factory with a senior manager in the 1950s. The factory was experimenting with robots performing manufacturing tasks.

> *Manager:*   *"How are you going to get the robots to pay union dues?"*
>
> *Union Boss:*   *"How are you going to get the robots to buy cars?"*

So, how are we affected when our work is impacted by robots or mismanagement or bad luck? In 2008, the Economic Journal published a study by Clark, Diener, Georgellis and Lucas. They followed 130,000 people over decades looking at lags and leads in the impact of life events. They asked, "Do individuals tend to return to some baseline level of well-being after life and labour market events?" They found, "Although the strongest life satisfaction effect is often at the time of the event, we find significant lag and lead effects. We cannot reject the hypothesis of complete adaptation to marriage, divorce, widowhood, birth of child and layoff. However, there is little evidence of adaptation to unemployment for men. Men are somewhat more affected by labour market events (unemployment and layoffs) than are women but in general the patterns of anticipation and adaptation are remarkably similar by sex."

They looked at major life events and how we bounced back from the knocks of the negative ones. The death of a spouse is a tough one but the longest negative impact on wellbeing, perhaps permanent, comes from *long-term unemployment.*

They don't just lose income with the poor health effects of that but they lose self worth and identity. People, especially men, who are carefree, undependable and unambitious in childhood, <u>and</u> have unsuccessful careers, have terrible mortality rates.

John Holland's Theory of Career Choice (RIASEC) maintains that in choosing a career, people prefer jobs where they can be around others who are like them. They search for environments that will let them use their skills and abilities, and express their attitudes and values, while taking on enjoyable problems and roles. Behaviour is determined by an interaction between personality and environment. He identified six types:

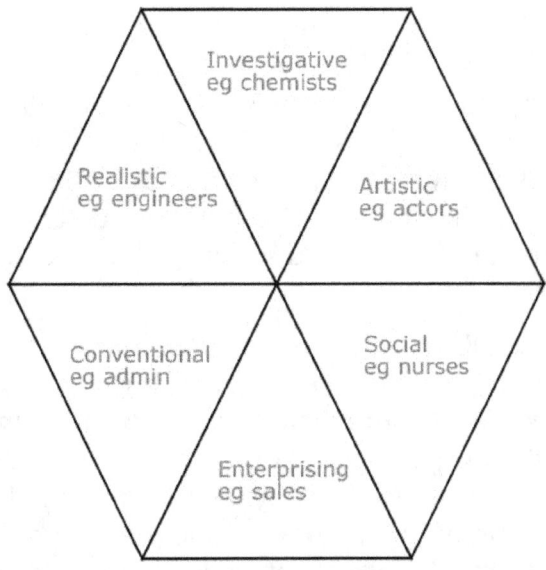

Mismatches in personality and career path does heighten risk of poor health and mortality but that risk is significantly lowered by a *productive perseverance*, a sense of mastery and accomplishment. These happen to be fundamental drivers of employee engagement. My last book 'The Brain-Based Boss' is a resource for employers trying to create a work environment that would allow their workers to be engaged. Engagement is the application of discretionary effort – people doing more than they have to because they choose to. There is ample evidence that engaged workplaces have higher productivity, revenue and profitability. That's great for the boss but what about non bosses? Why should they want to be engaged? Well, how about living a longer and more meaningful life?

Having a long commute sucks but did you realise how unhappy it could make you? Many voluntary conditions don't affect our happiness in the long-term because we acclimate to them. People never get used to their daily grind driving to work because sometimes the traffic is terrible and sometimes it isn't. Harvard psychologist

Daniel Gilbert says, "Driving in traffic is a different kind of hell every day." We rationalise this to ourselves and the family we don't see as often as we'd like by looking at our bigger house or higher salary. These rationalisations don't work. Swiss economists researched the effect of commuting on happiness and observed that such factors could not make up for the despair caused by a long commute.

The 10,000 hours thing has been done to death and back. The original piece of research by K. Anders Ericsson discovered much more than expertise requires an average of 10,000 hours of deliberate practice. In looking at the highest performers across many and varied fields, yes, a focused type of practice over time was critical but two other factors do not get enough attention. The highest performers get enough sleep and they do their 'work' in short productive bursts. Typically, these would be no more than ninety minutes. Not many jobs lend themselves to that but if we're genuinely interested in results rather than just cranking out hours at a desk, it's a provocative idea.

Remember back to this book's section on 'Moving.' Having a desk job can double your chances of contracting cardiovascular disease. Sitting is a big factor behind that problem. Here are just some of the downsides of prolonged periods of being motionless:

- Shuts off electrical activity in your large leg muscles,
- Calorie burning in your body drops to one per minute,
- Production of your fat-breaking enzymes drops by 90%,

- Two hours of sitting drops your good cholesterol levels by 20%.

Maybe you should be reading this book standing up?

One technique I'm a fan of these days is the 'Walking Meeting.' I've read of various companies that have meetings in rooms with no chairs. Their motivation, or more accurately – their boss's motivation, was to have more efficient meetings. The unintended upside is health! The Walking Meeting is self explanatory. I used to work for a City Council and I can imagine how much more efficient and pleasant experiences Council meetings would have been if we'd been strolling around Lake Pupuke. Quite aside from the health benefits and efficiencies, it might've reduced the length of some of the monologues.

Joking aside, the best conversations that took place in my experience as a Manager for that Council were the ones that took place in the field. Politicians, officers and residents would show up at the site of the building / pothole / proposed bus stop or wherever. Standing, walking, pointing, arguing etc was made all the more purposeful and productive not just because of the location in the real world but because *of the movement*. It literally ups everyone's energy levels which positively impacts creative thinking, attitudes and productivity. Things get done and you <u>feel</u> like things are getting done. You do not feel like that in a meeting room on your butt and that feeling drives negative physiological consequences.

"I don't want to achieve immortality through my work, I want to achieve it by not dying." – Woody Allen

6.1

Engage

Here's my quick definition of employee engagement – the application of discretionary effort. If we do more at work than we have to because we choose to (for whatever reason), that's externally observable and evidence that we are engaged in our work. Forget surveys where we tick boxes or mark numbers on a scale indicating what we think we remember we feel. There's no substitute for direct observation and it is our behaviour that always reveals us, despite what we may say or think we feel.

My previous book 'The Brain-Based Boss' provided loads of tips on how to create a workplace that is conducive to creating and maintaining motivation and engagement amongst teams. The benefits are proven for productivity, revenue and profitability. In this book, I'm looking more specially at the benefits to ourselves if we're engaged. If we do more than just show up, punch a clock and consume oxygen at work, how can it lead us to a longer, better and more productive and purposeful life?

Google has a policy that 20% of their staff's time is autonomous. They can work on projects of their own choosing. A couple of products that fell out of that policy were Google Sky and Gmail. Lazlo Bock, their Senior Vice President of People Operations commented, "When people at Google talk about what they like, this is one of the things they talk about. It's culturally important. Knowing that it exists causes people to feel more free."

Elizabeth Brondolo at St Johns University studied a group of parking wardens. Theirs is an inherently stressful job. They found that those workers with effective colleague support experienced less blood pressure spikes at times of high stress and lower retention of stress hormones. These benefits are not just psychological but physiological.

Chad Higgins from the University of Washington and Timothy Judge from the University of Florida analysed the factors behind why people got hired. Not what the hirers said were the factors but what really drove their decisions. The number one factor was... *likeability*. This book has already covered the health and longevity benefits of being likeable and socially active. It's also behind getting you the job and that promotion. And, if you're self employed, that's how you make sales, regardless of what you're selling. (And, if you're self employed, what you're selling is YOU!)

So to what extent, if you're engaged in your work, does this benefit you physically, mentally and socially?

In 2007, Elianne van Steenburgen and Naomi Ellemers looked at what they refer to as the 'work-family interface' and identified the benefits for both the employee and employer if work and family facilitate each other. Workers motivated to work by their families were measured to have lower cholesterol levels, a leaner body mass index and better physical stamina. Obviously this means they're more productive and less absent for the employer but also they're healthier for themselves.

Many employee wellness programmes offer free services such as five minute shoulder rubs in office workers' chairs from professional masseurs. Apart from the nice-to-have warm-fuzzy feeling, we've already covered the benefits of this in the earlier section on Touch. Not only is physical tension lessened in the area massaged but the act of touching and the ensuing spike in Oxytocin raises the sense of trust, honesty and helpfulness.

Christina Maslach in 2003 defined job burnout as a psychological syndrome resulting from a person-job misfit that involves exhaustion, cynicism and detachment from the job and a sense of ineffectiveness. To some extent, it is like being depressed about work and having little energy and enthusiasm for the job. Burnout can be divided into the following three components. *Emotional exhaustion* is the feeling of fatigue and tiredness at work. *Depersonalisation* is the development of a cynical and uncaring feeling towards others. *Reduced personal accomplishment* is when an employee feels that they are not accomplishing anything worthwhile.

It is well documented, according to the Irish Journal of Psychology, that the consequences of burnout include ill health, absenteeism and poor performance. Poor performance leads to fewer promotions and pay rises which mean less money which means, well, you know what that means. A track record of ill health, absenteeism and poor performance lowers your chances of scoring a different or better job in which you might become engaged.

Smart bosses know this and can see the mutual benefits of an engaged workforce. For the boss there is productivity improvement, increased revenues and more profit. The quid pro quo for those doing the work is greater chances for advancement, promotion, pay rises, as well as a healthier and happier life with some sense of meaning and achievement.

One survey of employers found a considerable intention to increase spending on employee wellness programmes over the next two years with 77% stating that they would increase or considerably increase spending. They don't see it as much a cost as an investment with a tangible return. So, it doesn't matter what your job is, if you're genuinely engaged in it, you're personally better off for it. We might live to work but that work helps us live.

6.2

Retire

A couple of years ago, we threw ourselves and our kids in a campervan and did a lap around New Zealand's South Island. One stop was a couple of days in Queenstown at a holiday park. Parked next to us was a retired couple from England. They were a hoot and a half. In conversation one morning, the woman said that they were touring the world "spending their kids' inheritance." My kids learned the meaning of the word 'inheritance' that day and I learned a different meaning of the word 'retirement.'

Japanese wives have a term for their retired husbands – Nure Ochiba. Literally translated, it means 'wet leaves.' Because, like wet leaves, they just hang around, get under your feet and aren't really doing anything useful. Less kind still is the term Sodai Gomi, 'inconvenient rubbish.' It was originally meant for items that you put out on the street for collection in what my City Council calls Inorganic Collection week. You keep banging your leg on it as you walk past and the wind just blows it about messing up the place. There's an old wives' saying about husbands, "I married him for life but not for lunch."

A New Zealand bank ran an advertising campaign for one of their retirement savings products with a catchy jingle, sarcastically called, 'I'm gonna work til I die.' The underlying assumption was that working was a bad thing done solely for income and less work was better. If that's true for you, then I'm very sorry. I want to write and talk about work in a broader sense. Not 'work' in the pejorative sense of having to show up, clock on and do something for someone else that we'd rather not be doing solely for a wage. The work I'm talking about covers our activities that have meaning and purpose and help keep us active, connected, mindful and *alive*. You'd be crazy to want to retire from that. A 2013 study by Hernaes, Markussen, Piggott and Vestad of data on the entire population of Norway found that shifting retirement ages had no impact on mortality on average. Other studies have found it can have specific effects. In fact, many people in some professions that have dedicated themselves to a particular career and even totally identified themselves via it, have a terrible mortality rate following retirement. In 2012, Kuhn, Wuellrich and Zweimuller found that, for men, one additional year of early retirement causes an increase in the risk of premature death by 2.4%. And that was in blue collar jobs, not bank managers. The study showed that for every extra year of early retirement, workers lost about two months of life expectancy.

The authors suggest it might be something as simple as having too much time on their hands and using those idle hands to sit, smoke and consume alcohol excessively – things which equivalently retired women tend not to do. There's also the loss of purposefulness. A 2005 survey conducted by Harris Interactive found different age groups had different levels of agreement with the statement "A good deal of my pride comes from my work and career":

- Over 55 years old 59%
- 35-54 years old 48%
- 18-34 years old 37%

Boston College's Centre for Aging and Workplace Flexibility found that people stayed on formal past retirement age for the money but there other primary reasons are:

- I enjoy the job 76%
- I like being productive & helping others 68%
- It makes me feel useful 66%

Their report says older workers who have responsibilities for dependent family members are less likely to retire and withdraw from the labour force. 21% of workers who expect to work during their "retirement" years anticipate making this decision so that they can help to support children or other family members

If we are supposed to leave high school at age 18 and retire at age 65, yet we're living to 80, is it realistic or desirable to spend 25% of our adult lives in this limbo state called 'retirement'? When high school was a machine to prepare most of us for terrible jobs of boredom and labour that wore us down, then retirement was probably a good thing. A rest well earned. This industrial-age meets welfare-state timeline looks like this:

EDUCATION – WORK - RETIREMENT

The upside of the above traditional approach is certainty and stability. People like that and Governments like that. It enables us to plan, collectively and individually. The problem is that the world that supported that timeline no longer exists. Personally, I am seeing a lot more people's lives reflecting the timeline below and it is what I want for myself:

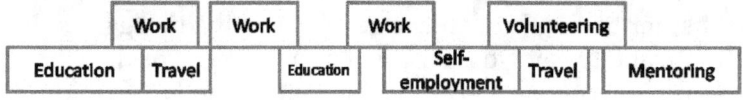

Even this is just indicative as it is a highly personal choice-based approach. You could throw in any number of additional time blocks – 'periodic retirements', sabbaticals, 'phased retirement.' Years ago, Charles Handy wrote of 'Portfolio Lifestyles' and that's what I've been aspiring to. This DIY-jigsaw approach to our personal career timelines is uncertain, unstable and messy. It's actually unlikely to be as simple as the example I have used. It probably won't be linear or flat. There is no pre-defined end point. I don't like the concept of an end point in my timeline (although I am more than accepting that there will be an end point.) I want 'purpose points' and lots of them. Technology, industrialisation and mass-consumerism have given us an age of abundance and choice (if you live in the right countries.) The abundance is killing many of us but it is that power of choice that will save those of us with the courage to use it.

New Zealand Census data shows 40% of 65 to 69-year-olds and 21% of 70 to 74-year olds were in fulltime or part-time employment in 2013. Grey Power president Roy Reid said there were several factors in the choice to keep working. "The first one is definitely financial. Secondly, there are people who reach the age of 65 and are fit and well and quite capable of work and do choose to carry on. A lot of them go part-time, maybe four days' work a week." A report issued by the Ministry of Social Development said a labour and skills shortage was a major factor in increasing employment levels for over 65s, which have been on the rise since 2002.

According to data from the U.S. Bureau of Labour Statistics, 42% of American workers aged 65 and older are running an established small business, 9% own a business that's less than 3.5 years old, and 11% own a fledgling new business. So, 62% of older 'workers' aren't employees, they're self-employed. Whether this is through choice or necessity, it suggests that if you want to set yourself up for a better working life and retirement on your terms, you need to open your mind to the prospect of some form of entrepreneurship. 26% of workers aged over 65 said they planned to launch a business. Ray Kroc started McDonalds when he was 52.

The Kauffman Index of Entrepreneurial Activity noted that of new entrepreneurs in 2011:

- 21% were aged 55 to 64, up from 14% in 1996

- 28% were aged 45 to 54, up from 24%

- 22% were aged 35-44, down from 27

- 29% were aged 20 to 34, down from 35%

The ones who succeed leverage their social capital, not just their investment capital. We've all got the friend with the great idea or ideas who never gets anything done. In entrepreneurship, it's never the idea, it's the execution. Whatever your age is right now, you'd better put some effort into developing your social capital – your network of connections. Once again, it's your connectivity to the rescue. It's not only the number one driver of your health and longevity, it's the means by which you can help fund that longer and healthier life.

How can you extend your network? The next section on volunteering can help – give a little to get a lot.

6.3

Volunteer

"Live as if you were to die tomorrow; learn as if you were to live forever." – Mahatma Gandhi

Thomas Glass ran a study I referred to earlier about the positive impact of socializing for our health and longevity. The Harvard Gazette reports he is now working with a group from Johns Hopkins University in Baltimore on a project to put seniors into inner-city elementary schools. The oldsters work with children who need more help developmentally than most teachers have time to give. "We are measuring the impact on both the seniors and the kids," Glass says. "So far the program, called the Experience Corps, looks promising.

"By helping to keep the faucet of social engagement running for elders," Glass continues, "society taps into a huge source of skill and experience. In return, older people receive the kind of meaning and purpose in their lives that buffers them from physical and cognitive deterioration."

Meaning and purpose keep us healthier and alive longer and not just in our senior years. A disproportionate amount of volunteering is done by older folk. In my own careers, I've come across several groups run by volunteer retirees. The research suggests more of us pre-retirees and those just starting out could glean a lot of benefits from volunteering and not just warm fuzzy feelings.

At one stage in the work-skills programme I mentioned earlier in conjunction with a power company, Iwi and Ministry of Social Development, the participants were drafting their CVs. All were long-term unemployed and they ranged in age from 20 to 60. One woman sat staring at her computer screen for ages, looking more lost than lost in thought. She lamented that she had no skills to write down. Within three questions, I heard about how she'd been secretary at her local rugby league club for years. She'd drafted their constitution. She'd negotiated the lease on the land their club was on. She organised and ran multiple fundraising events and tournaments. She had plenty of skills but what she lacked was a mindset to recognise them.

She'd never considered her volunteering as secretary to be work. Initially, she had signed up because her kids were players at the club but even after they grew up and left town, she stayed on. Many of the intangibles that employed people got, she got from her volunteering role. But it wasn't all one-way-traffic, she got something back in return. It was a collection of practical and useful returns, not just a glow of altruism.

Benefits include:

- New transferable skills,
- Development of existing skills,
- Proving the application of your skills,
- Exposure to new people,
- Exposure to change,
- A sense of purpose,
- Involvement with people with a shared passion,
- Feedback that what you do matters,
- Connection with your community,
- Flesh our your CV,
- Gain new perspectives to take back to work and family,

- Networking opportunities for new jobs & business opportunities,

- Setting a positive example to your family,

- Gaining or retaining the respect of your family & yourself during periods of unemployment or retirement.

Are these skills genuinely transferable?

- 73% of employers would choose someone with volunteering experience over someone without if skill levels were comparable otherwise,

- 94% of employers believe that skills and experience gained during volunteering are valid in the paid workforce,

- 94% of employees with volunteering experience say that their volunteering has contributed to them getting their first job, an improved salary, or a promotion.

The health, longevity and life quality benefits we get from the right kind of work need not come from paying job. Volunteering may seem like a selfless act but it could do you and your family the world of good.

6.4

Paths

"Man sacrifices his health in order to make money. Then he sacrifices money to recuperate his health. And then he is so anxious about the future that he does not enjoy the present; the result being that he does not live in the present or the future; he lives as if he is never going to die, and then he dies having never really lived." – Dalai Lama

When asked if they like what they do each day, only 20% of people answer yes.

Consider the wishful thinking behind people's choice to pay for a swimming pool to be installed at their home and the ongoing maintenance costs versus the reality. They imagine life will be a constant whirl of pool parties, barbecues and aquatic adventure and frivolity. The vast majority of times, pool buyers sit in traffic going to and from jobs they dislike to fund pools that they don't have the time or energy to enjoy. Dunn and Norton have a fantastic technique for addressing this 'pool paradox' – Think about Tuesday. The next time you're pondering a major purchase, think back to the reality of last Tuesday. Would you or your friends and family have been able to enjoy the use of that item in the time and circumstances that existed last Tuesday? How much time, energy and inclination were available after school, work, chores, homework, commitments, dinner and so forth. How was the weather? Not every day is like those perfect summer Saturdays of your memory or your imagination (or your imagination's memory.) Most days are like last Tuesday.

Charles Handy wrote of work as a number of portfolios from which to choose – paid work, gift work, study work and home work. Re-chunk your time.

Choice architecture is a label applied to how we can guide behaviour through adapting the physical environment. Doors in public buildings often have signs on them saying 'push' or 'pull'. Despite these signs you often see people pulling a 'push' door or pushing a 'pull' door. I've done that. Sometimes you'll hurt a muscle. Always you'll hurt your pride. Choice Architecture dictates that a push door should be obviously pushable. It shouldn't have a handle to pull.

My favourite example of behaviour change driven through environmental design was Ade Kieboom's urinal fly at an airport in the Netherlands. They reduced cleaning costs by 80% via having small images of flies etched into the urinals. A clever idea that proved effective and has been copied the world over.

The choices made by children in school cafeterias can be affected by the physical placement of the food choices. Simple geographic proximity is a powerful thing. A study showed that having the healthier choices in prime locations was a more effective long-term behaviour shifter than nanny state prohibitions.

We need money. Gotta pay the bills. But if your bills are paid, money can taint your enjoyment of the things and experiences you do have. Even the thought of money can do that. Here's a 2-step experiment for you.

1. How many hours do you work a week? How many weeks did you work last year? How much did you earn last year? Work out what your time is worth by dividing your annual income by the hours you worked in that year.

2. Go and listen to your favourite song for its entire length.

Studies on people doing simple activities like the one above have shown that people experience reduced enjoyment. Their favourite song has less appeal to them once they've been primed to perceive listening to it as a waste of valuable time. We do this to ourselves all the time.

It can be flipped and turned to our advantage. My brother-in-law flies planes. During his learning days, he needed to get his hours up and, when you're a civilian and non-movie star, that costs a lot of money. He then re-framed all other uses of his money in terms of how many flying hours he'd be sacrificing if he spent it. Maybe he should get a new pair of shoes? Is it worth the loss of a flying hour? It worked for him. (Though, I suspect my sister got a tad jaded about it.)

6.5

Plans and Goals

Here's an excerpt about goals from my 2008 book 'The Guide: How to Kiss, Get A Job & Other Stuff You Need To Know.'

To be effective, goals need to be written with a lot of thought and SMART personal meaning.

- **S**pecific ('Lose weight' or 'Save money' is too vague.)

- **M**easurable

- **A**spirational (They need to stretch and challenge you. Any goal that aims for you to stay the same ain't worth having.)

- **R**ealistic (Brad Pitt or Jennifer Lopez might not be out of your league but Brad Pitt <u>and</u> Jennifer Lopez at the same time definitely are.)

- **T**imed

Examples of SMART Goals:

By 31 December 2020, my weight will be in the range 85-90kg.

By 30 June 2021, I will have $5000 in my savings account for my Costa Rican scuba adventure holiday.

During 2020, I will have had three dinner parties at my house at which I will have met at least three new friends.

The first and third Fridays of every month will be, without exception, reserved for alone-time for my partner and me for a night on the town.

Stick on some pictures to bring those goals alive. It's the pictures that supply the 'why' and remind you why each goal is important. Five thousand dollars is in itself nothing but a means to an end. What's the end-game for you? If it's a tropical scuba adventure, don't paste a picture of a moneybag, paste a picture of a coral reef or something that flicks your bic. Post your illustrated goal grid on your wall where you'll see it every day. Tell others about it.

It's in our nature to do things that provide the most immediate reward. It's best to find short-term incentives that are consistent with our long-term objectives. If you're at a crossroads for lunch and one option is a cheeseburger, the prospect of obesity is not an immediately effective disincentive. One cheeseburger won't make you obese and that potential obesity is in the future. The 'fat hangover' the cheeseburger will give you might be a disincentive. It is in the immediate future and is definite. You will feel sluggish and blah and if you need to be on your game after lunch then that might sway your behaviour. It's more likely to be successful than worrying about your future older self. You don't know that person nor really care about them. Not as much as you care about special sauce.

The Nicoyan Costa Ricans have a phrase, "Plan de vida." A plan for life. For many of these long-living folk, that plan doesn't just plan for both work and family, it integrates them. Although, historically this was out of economic necessity, these days the benefits are evident.

It's not just big life plans that drive behaviour with meaning and purpose. The very act of measuring anything can drive improvement in that activity. Common for years now in workplaces have been wellness programmes like 10,000 steps handing out pedometers. The devices themselves create a focus and it is focus that often drives behaviour. Add in the social impact of others with the same devices and the same focus and the effect is magnified. Some newer devices like the range from FitBit and their associated smartphone apps have 'badges' and 'points' which again drive a sense of community, shared effort and social norming.

My daughter's name is Isabel and that's how we spell it. There's an app called *Isabel* which allows users to self-diagnose. You can get an app to run an EKG on yourself or friends. Always handy at a party.

Living until 90 or saving for retirement are not great goals as they are written. The former is in the future and, as such, research strongly shows that it is not an effective motivator as we face daily decisions. We make over 200 choices a day to do with food alone. The latter is too vague – saving how much and by when would make it a better goal. The most effective approach is to self-identify a collection of near-term motivators that mean something to you right now and that will push you the right way when your brain faces a decision that your body can't be trusted on. Place constant reminders of those motivators around you at home, work and in the car.

One example of such a near-term motivator might be your wish to have better quality interactions with your family. Coming home stressed, tired, unhappy and funked up with junk food, inactivity and poor sleep do not make for an awesome evening of being a great parent or partner.

Maybe you aspire to political leadership? A 2013 study by White, Kendrick and Neuberg at the Psychology Department at Arizona State University found that voters prefer healthier-looking candidates and the more unhealthy the region, the greater the preference for healthier-looking candidates. So, by taking up the twelve controls, you not only better your odds of living longer and better, you will also look like you will, which will subconsciously boost others' opinion of you.

(I can recall two recent U.S. elections where dead candidates won, having died after they submitted their entry into the race. I assume they submitted really healthy looking photos?)

LOVE

Love might seem out of place or superfluous in a book about adding 10 years to your productive life but, as I've tried to repeatedly emphasise, living longer for its own sake is pointless and motivates few. Many of the controls I've highlighted in this book are pretty simple but might take a bit of work, sacrifice and change. There needs to be a reason for most of us to work, sacrifice or change.

Money might be a reason but money is merely a medium of exchange with which we acquire what we want and, apart from that top 1% we keep hearing about, what we're exchanging that money for is food, shelter and so forth for the ones we love. Or things that we hope will attract someone who might love us.

There has to be a point. People need to have meaning and we'll make it up if it doesn't exist.

Be it love of your community or of your immediate family, that's probably why we do what we do and why we'd like to do it better and for longer.

7.1

Self

In his book 'Thrive', Dan Buettner recommends strategies for happiness across six inter-related 'Thrive centres' derived from lessons learned in the happiest places on Earth. (None of which were Disneyland.)

1. Community

- Community spaces like parks
- Quiet surroundings
- Walking distance
- Safety

2. Workplace

- The right job (Seek a better boss)
- Avoid long commutes
- Don't skip vacations

3. Social Life

- Upgrade your social network
- Create your own group of mutually committed friends
- Marry the right person

4. Financial Life

- Automate savings plans
- Avoid debt

5. Home

- Design a 'flow' room to chill in
- Garden

Optimise your bedroom for sleep

6. Self

- Have a personal mission statement
- Develop your people skills
- Volunteer

Try his 'True Happiness Test' at
http://apps.bluezones.com/happiness/ (I got a B+.)

Looking after yourself can have unexpected positive consequences. Lan Nguyen Chaplin and Deborah Roedder John did studies that showed that low self esteem leads to materialistic urges. Everything you ever suspected about drivers of expensive status cars you now know to be true.

Fritz Strack did a fun experiment in 1988 that you can try whilst reading this book. The health benefits of happiness get triggered by the oddest things. If your body smiles, your brain assumes that you're happy and releases all that happiness hormone juice. The smile need not be genuine. It should be and it's better if it is but, meanwhile, try this. Put a pencil between your teeth and don't let your lips tough the pencil. The same muscles required to do that are your smiling muscles.

Subsequent research by Robert Soussignan in 2002 demonstrated that smiling will accentuate a positive emotional experience, but will have no effect on a negative experience.

7.2

Friends

"Relationships come and go but friends
are for life." – Somebody that I used to know

The British Medical Journal in August 1999 published a study of 3000 people aged over 65 that they followed for 13 years. The study tracked their participation in activities such as swimming, walking, shopping, volunteer work, social group activities and so forth. It transpires that social engagement is the best medicine.

Thomas Glass at Harvard's School of Public Health studied 2761 people over 13 years and their socialising, concluding that it could increase longevity by 20%. As the Harvard Gazette put it, "Scientists are always coming up with ways for older people to live healthier and longer lives, such as doing exercises they can't or don't want to do. Now, researchers have found an easier way: people 65 years and older can extend their lives by doing things that are easy and enjoyable, like going to church or movies, shopping, gardening, and even playing bingo."

"Such activities should not replace exercise," Glass cautions, "but exclusive emphasis on exercise may be overly narrow. It is clear from our study that **social engagement can have as much effect on prolonging life as fitness activities**." The smart move at whatever age is to double up and participate in exercise-based social activities. Notice now the massive increase in the popularity of group sessions at gyms and with personal trainers. It's not just another way for gyms to charge multiple people at once instead of a single-customer personal training session. The evidence suggests you might get as much benefit from the interaction as from the exertion. The exercises might change by the time you're 70 but the social benefits remain the same.

The Harvard Gazette went on to report that Glass admits he doesn't know precisely why. However, he believes that keeping social and busy "evokes changes in the brain that protect against cognitive decline. This, in turn, influences physical processes regulated by the brain such as cellular immunity or mobilizing the body's defences against disease."

In other research, Glass and two colleagues tracked the effect of social disengagement on 2,812 people 65 years and older for 12 years. They found the odds of experiencing cognitive decline were approximately twice as great in those reporting no social ties than in those who had frequent contact with relatives and friends, attended religious services, or participated in regular social activities.

Another study revealed that rats who sustain brain injury and who socialize and have fun during recovery do much better than those who are socially isolated, even when both groups receive optimum physical care. This is why I'm not a scientist - I don't know what rats do for fun.

We get influenced by the habits of our friends. We get a sense of belonging, purpose and self worth. It also works the other way though. For example, 56% of people trying to eat healthily will eat crap to avoid insulting a host, boss, client or family member. 51% will eat crap to fit in with the group. So, it pays to choose our friends wisely and 'audit' your ongoing value to each other.

If you have a best friend at work, you are seven times more likely to feel engaged in your job.

Friends have a powerful social influence. For one obvious example, be observant the next time you're out for dinner with a group of friends and you get to that point of the evening when the waiter or waitress shows up and asks, "Would anyone like to see the dessert menu?" I'd gotten into the habit of saying something witty about just having a look, or at least something as witty as I was capable of after however much wine had entered my system before dessert. (ie most of it.) Now, I shut up and watch. You should too. The most common group dynamic when that question is asked is a fleeting flurry of eye contact amongst all members of the table. Each member of the group is determining their response to the question based on their perception of the likely reaction of everyone else. Again, the first person to react over-influences the subsequent responses of everyone else.

The restaurants know this. It is in their interest to sell more desserts and to keep you drinking the higher profit margin drinks, and if you stay for dessert, you'll be there longer and you'll get more drinks. Again, observe the waiter or waitress. They do not just ask the general group of people at the table a question. The question is directed at the person they think is most likely to answer, "Yes." Just like lions hunting gazelles, the restaurants prey on the weakest member of the herd. And, in your group of friends, you all know who that is. If you don't, it's you.

Psychological priming is where a behaviour can be steered by exposure to a previous stimulus. Give two groups of research participants free cookies while filling in a fake quiz but expose one group to the smell of cleaning products and you'll find the clean smell-primed group tidies up their crumbs and plates twice as often. The social influence of friends and menu choices is a form of priming. But priming doesn't work if you know it is happening. So, armed with this knowledge, take a bit more control over what you consume and spend. Tell your friends. That's what friends are for.

In a very recent piece of research, 'Bad Boys: The Effect of Criminal Identity on Dishonesty,' Alain Cohn, Michel Andre Marechal, and Thomas Noll reveal a potential negative application of priming effects that you and I might be able to flip and use with our friends to more positive ends. In a maximum security prison they had prisoners privately toss coins and then say how many times the coin landed heads. The more heads turned up, the more money the prisoners got paid. The researchers couldn't tell if any single prisoner was honest or dishonest but they did know that on average heads comes up half the time, so they can assess in aggregate how much lying there is. Before the study, they had half the prisoners answer the question "What were you convicted for?" and the other half "How many hours per week do you watch television on average?" The result: 66% heads in the treatment where they ask about convictions and "only" 60% heads in the TV treatment. Being reminded or primed about their dishonesty drove greater dishonesty in their behaviour.

How dishonest are prisoners versus everyday people? When they play the same game with regular citizens, the coin supposedly comes up heads 56% of the time. Most people are also dishonest but less so than primed or unprimed prisoners.

Flipping this notion of priming, we need to find ways of subtly 'reminding' ourselves or our loved ones that we are the sort of person who behaves in ways that support us in boosting our healthy and productive lifestyles. This would vary from person to person and over time. One suggestion might be agreeing to exchange a daily text at an agreed time with a buddy. Nothing arduous, mentally taxing, syrupy or faux motivational – just some words about whatever it is you're trying to support each other on. Remind them that they are whatever they need to be. Routinise it and prioritise it.

A University of Virginia study looked at participants sent out to estimate the steepness of a hill before setting out to climb it with a weighted backpack. Half the participants had a friend with them and half did not. Those with friends guessed lower steepness levels and the longer the friendships with their climbing companions, the greater the underestimation of steepness. Having a friend with you not only lowers your stress levels as we've identified earlier, it makes the task ahead seem less foreboding. And we know how our perceptions and preconceptions can affect us physically.

Even if your buddy and you end up in a debate over things, that's not inherently bad. In fact, it is really only your good friends with whom you can genuinely argue and care about the meaning of the result. Arguments with friends stimulate the plasticity of the brain. Surround yourself with people with helpful values, not necessarily the same as yours. Identify your 'inner circle.' Be likeable. Create time and opportunities to be together.

If you want to broaden or replace your social circuit, here are some tips:

- Walk your dog (or child.) At least, they'll be good conversation starters,

- Work out,

- Do lunch,

- Accept the next 3 invitations you get regardless,

- Volunteer,

- Attend community events,

- Take classes,

- Fake a faith. (Faith is like sincerity, in that if you can fake that, you've got it made.)

Social isolation is a major risk factor. Having no friends or low-interaction friends is as bad as smoking 15 cigarettes a day, as dangerous as being an alcoholic and twice as harmful as obesity. In a six-year study of 736 middle-age Swedish men, attachment to a single person didn't appear to affect the risk of heart attack and fatal coronary heart disease, but having friendships did. Only smoking was as important a risk factor as lack of social support.

The New York Times reported on some sub-research by a pair of social scientists named Nicholas Christakis and James Fowler using the information collected over the years by the Framingham Heart Study. Founded in 1948 by the National Heart Institute, the study follows more than 15,000 Framingham residents and their descendants, bringing them in to a doctor's office every four years, on average, for a comprehensive physical. By analysing the Framingham data, Christakis and Fowler say, they have for the first time found some solid basis for a potentially powerful theory in epidemiology: that good behaviours, like quitting smoking or staying slender or being happy, pass from friend to friend almost as if they were contagious viruses. The Framingham participants, the data suggested, influence each another's health just by socializing. And the same was true of bad behaviours — clusters of friends appeared to "infect" each other with obesity, unhappiness and smoking. Staying healthy isn't just a matter of your genes and your diet, it seems. Good health is also a product, in part, of your sheer proximity to other healthy people.

You don't need a lot of friends but you do need the right ones.

So next time you suggest to someone that you become 'friends with benefits', be sure to stress that you mean *health* benefits...

> *"Anybody can sympathise with the*
> *sufferings of a friend, but it requires a very*
> *fine nature to sympathise with a friend's*
> *success." – Oscar Wilde*

7.3

Partner(s)

"Before you get married, ask yourself: Is this the person you want to watch stare at their phone for the rest of your life?" – Julius Sharpe

Married men live ten years longer than single men and married women live four years longer than single women. Divorce is not healthy at all. Though I might observe that for many couples, divorce might be less unhealthy than staying together.

Beyond the chemical and hormonal cocktail our brains choose to interpret as love, the practice of maintaining a loving monogamous relationship is a set of skills that can be learned and needs to be practised and applied. That's yet another set of small choices we can make every day that we might like to add to our ever-increasing list of tiny habits.

Here is a menu of love-supportive behaviours:

- Accept their love,
- Accept them as they are,
- Accept them growing,
- Accept that people are different,
- Remain curious,
- Be supportive,

- Always build them up,

- Talk,

- Don't make comparisons,

- Let go of negativity,

- Plenty of physical contact,

- Sex (Duh),

- Do special things often,

- Take care of them,

- Think of terms of 'us' (Listen to your words.)

A 2003 study for the University of North Carolina by Karen Grewen and Kathleen Light looked at couples' interactions and physical health impacts. They had two groups of couples and baseline measurements were taken of heart rate and blood pressure. One group's couples held hands, watched a short romantic video and engaged in a twenty second embrace. The other group did not. Everyone was then compelled to do some short unprepared public speaking which is pretty stressful for most people. They all had their heart rate and blood pressure monitored before, throughout and after their speech. The couples who had experienced the hand holding etc had increases in heart rate and blood pressure due to the stress of the speech but significantly less so than the other group.

We're all familiar with life cycles. The seasons of the year – Winter, Spring, Summer, Autumn and back to Winter again. (Relationships between younger and older people are sometimes referred to as a 'Spring and Autumn' relationship, although they are more often referred to as 'ickky.') Marketing academics are convinced products have a life cycle. They write about customer relationship life cycles. The same is true of romantic relationships. We instinctively know this. There is something exciting yet scary about that special someone in the early stages. You discover what turns them on. You discover what turns them off. You discover that what you thought turned them on actually turns them off. There's risk and passion. But, even if it lasts a long time, it doesn't last. A sense of familiarity creeps in which isn't inherently bad; it's just different.

Relationships also undergo change over time, quite apart from any changes occurring to the individuals within the relationship. That change can happen to you or you can make it happen – with good reason.

Sigmoid Curves – Reinventing the Relationship

The performance of anything requires maintenance, be it a car, a company or a relationship, but more than just maintenance in the sense of care or upkeep. So many of us keep doing what we're doing – with our diet, our jobs, our relationships. Only when something goes wrong do we react. Change is going to occur. We can wait and react and be victims to that change or we can be proactive, take charge and control our destiny.

The notion of the sigmoid curve from organisational performance as described below by Charles Handy is scarily applicable to relationships.

"The first of the curves represents a normal life cycle of anything...: a period of learning or investment, in which inputs exceed outputs, followed by steady growth that inevitably one day peaks and turns into decline. The only variable is the length of the curve, the time it takes to reach the various points on the curve. The only way to prolong the life of the body in question, be it an organization or even a career, is to start a second curve. But to allow time and resources for the initial period of learning and investment, that second curve has to start before the first one peaks. You then encounter the paradox of success -- when things

are going well, there seems to be no reason to change. Reluctance to change ultimately turns success into failure."

So, the point of this is that you need to re-invent the relationship just as things are almost at their best. By anticipating the inevitable decline you can prevent it. It is as though you are entering another relationship but with the same person, garnering all those special vibes of a new fling but without having to change address or buy a secret pre-pay cellphone to conduct a clandestine affair.

Just remember – every time you feel as happy as you can be, it won't last – unless you do something about it.

7.4

Family

George Vaillant is the director of a 72-year study of the lives of 268 men. In an interview in the March 2008 newsletter to the Grant Study subjects, Vaillant was asked, "What have you learned from the Grant Study men?" Vaillant's response: "That the only thing that really matters in life are your relationships to other people." He shared insights of the study with Joshua Wolf Shenk at The Atlantic on how the men's social connections made a difference to their overall happiness: The men's relationships at age 47, he found, predicted late-life adjustment better than almost any other variable. Good sibling relationships seem especially powerful: 93 percent of the men who were thriving at age 65 had been close to a brother or sister when younger.

I started this book talking about why you should care about living longer, better and more productively. A big part of that is to do with family. We will never live forever but, to a degree, we can via our families. So, I think it fitting that we close the loop by addressing this as a form of personal social investment.

We invest in all sorts of things. As nations we invest in infrastructure. As individuals, we need to invest in social capital. If you're a bit of a free market freak and your hackles start to raise at the touchy feely notion of investing in social capital, fret note, you can have selfish interests at the centre of this too.

There's the family you're born into and there is the family you make yourself as an adult. It might be the traditional Western stereotypical model of parents and a single generation of kids. It might be one of a wide variety of other models with multiple generations. Never mind the old chestnut about it taking a village to raise a child, it takes a bunch of people to support us in good health and productivity. If we don't have those people, we need to find them or make them, or else we'll suffer the consequences.

Family is down to luck and choices. A 2007 study in the *American Journal of Psychiatry* reported that men who had poor relationships with even one sibling before the age of 20 were significantly more likely to become depressed by the age of 50 than men who had gotten along with their siblings, quite separate of their relationship with their parents. Maybe sometimes they had siblings who were jerks, maybe sometimes they were jerks. The reasons are immaterial after a while. The effects and impacts are not. Just like your height which you got via genetics, you got some family as well. Sometimes the luck of it is that you got some unhelpful or even hurtful family. Go listen to an Eminem album for a while to get some perspective and a frame of reference. You might think you've married your soulmate and good on you if you think that but in terms of impact on your longevity, happiness and health, it's your siblings that rule. And 82% of people have siblings.

Remember earlier how I quoted Terman's longitudinal study that indicated health and longevity is most highly driven by people with conscientious personalities? If you've got siblings, check out the oldest. How conscientious are they? Research indicates that on average, oldest kids are the most conscientious. The youngest are the ones generally into at-risk behaviours which can result in accidents, illnesses and shorter, less productive lives.

Frank Sulloway is a Psychologist and a visiting scholar at the University of California at Berkeley. He is well known for his investigation of the effects of birth order. Birth order is one of the major factors driving sibling diversification. With their parents' solo attention in their earliest years, firstborns are often most expected to uphold family values and traditions and act as surrogate parents (especially oldest females), fostering the development of conscientiousness. By the time last-borns arrive, they have little to lose by rejecting expectations and taking risks. According to Sulloway, it's all very Darwinian. (Darwin was the 5th of 6 kids. Copernicus was the 4th of 4 and he took some risks. Probably thought he was the centre of the universe...)

I have two brothers and two sisters. I'm the fourth of five kids. Without getting into personal details that my family wouldn't appreciate, I'm pretty confident that we don't fit the birth order pattern but we do display marked diversity. And I reckon it's the middle one that has rebelliousness and non-conformity in spades. I have a son and a daughter. I'm not sure if I can objectively classify either as having large amounts of conscientiousness or risk-taking behaviours yet. I'm pretty safe mentioning them. One of them doesn't even read my books, even though my first two books were specifically dedicated to them. "Look, read to page 5, your name is on it!"

The magazine *Psychology Today* suggests that for siblings who are closest in age, "De-identification is most urgent, forcing siblings adjacent in the family constellation to develop opposing personality traits." Middle children are the ones to look out for too but for different reasons. "They receive less cumulative investment than do eldest and lastborn offspring," Sulloway says. And that explains why they go through life with lower self-esteem, feel more self-conscious, and often feel closer to friends than to parents.

A new study by researchers from Ohio State University suggests that growing up with siblings lays the foundation for healthy relationships later in life and might even lessen the likelihood of marital breakdown. Each sibling you have reduces your odds of a divorce by 2%. Arguably, this might be because as a youngster growing up with multiple points of view, differing opinions and competition for resources, you have to develop coping skills. These skills suit you for later life in other relationships, be they marriage, friends or professional relationships. Interestingly, only-children have a lower likelihood of ever getting married at all.

It's not all bad news for only-children though. A Swedish study found they did better academically and had a much greater chance of becoming university qualified. They can hang their degrees on their walls. There's space there, unoccupied by wedding photos.

So, again, if you haven't got any siblings, you need to find some people you can plug into that gap in your life as best you can as soon as you can. You don't have to but there are benefits if you can.

Western family units are shrinking and dispersing. Maybe we need to incentivise young families to live in older communities? Recently, I went through a few years of renting houses to live in in between owning them myself. In doing so, I moved around a few times and had quite a diversity of neighbours. Old folks are good. They're quiet and always around, so are great for the neighbourhood watch safety aspect. Kids are great for keeping active and energised. There is proven value in intergenerational diversity and connectivity. Listen to each other. Laugh with each other. Learn from each other.

Teenagers that cook, regardless of what they cook as teenagers, go on to eat more healthily as adults. Plan meals together well ahead of time so you have ingredients to hand. Plan the shopping around that meal plan.

Caring for your kids' health should start even before you conceive them. It's (hopefully) pretty common knowledge that pregnant women shouldn't smoke or drink alcohol during pregnancy. (Neither should the dads either of course. It's a team game guys!) Less well known is the long-term impact on babies of a mother's obesity. Pregnant women need to be encouraged to lose excess weight and quit smoking to avoid causing brain damage to their unborn children, according to a research team at Brigham and Women's Hospital in Boston. Led by Kiwi paediatric neurologist Terrie Inder, they use sophisticated imaging techniques to predict and manage the risk of disabilities for at-risk infants.

But if our own potential obesity is a sensitive issue, crazily it's even more sensitive if it's suggested to be a problem for our kids. Sarah Harvey reported in stuff.co.nz that more than 80 per cent of parents with overweight children do not know they are overweight and health professionals hold back from telling them because of the risk of getting parents' backs up, according to Rachael Taylor from Otago University's School of Medicine. They sought to find a way for parents to be safely told their child had weight problems. Taylor was part of a group of 11 researchers who screened 1500 children in Dunedin. They found parents responded positively to the use of a traffic-light system, where children were plotted as either green (OK) orange (some issues) or red (definite health issues).

You can create a health-supportive culture within your family through rituals and labels. Apart from the fibre in the stick, there is little value in eating a hot dog. Re-label that hot dog 'Shit On A Stick' and get it ingrained in your family. Notice how it affects demand for hot dogs. I doubt I'll get much traction in my house relabelling chocolate chip cookies as 'Cancer Discs.'

The evidence clearly shows that strong and effective familial ties and support add to the quality and quantity of your life. I also acknowledge that, for many people, it won't. It's up to you to do the maths in your head as to the potential benefits outweigh the grief if your family is hard work, abusive, parasitic, distant or otherwise non-supportive. Please do include in your equation your kids. Your mommy issues shouldn't impede the benefits they might derive from intergenerational connectivity.

The MacArthur Study of Successful Aging looked at 1189 people aged 70-79 over 7 years. They found families represented the highest degree of supportive social network. If you haven't got such a supportive family, you need to make one or create a substitute model with friends, colleagues or knit one out of wool. But you need one. The study does provide the proviso that family members need to be connected but independent and close, but not too close, geographically. They also note the values of family rituals like the Sunday lunch or movie outings and physical places where family is celebrated. Not literally a shrine but a wall of remembrance or similar for photos, trophies, mementos etc.

Maybe your family isn't a biological one but you've welded a facsimile together over time by choice. Regardless, ultimately this is where we find out why we want to live longer, more healthily and productively. The 'why' is the 'who' and the 'who' are your family.

Don't Just Know It... Do It!

"Why do people have to die?"

"To make life important."

Six Feet Under

I recently attended a special assembly at my kids' college. My son was getting an award for Physics. (Me, I'm happy that gravity, momentum and opposite and equal reactions exist but I'm not fussed about getting into too much more detail.) Midway through the event, one of the school's award-winning choirs took to the stage to perform. I really enjoyed it but I didn't fully understand it. Eventually, I worked out that it was in a foreign language and, even then, it took a while for me to get specific on which one. I didn't fully understand it and I didn't fully appreciate it. I just know that I enjoyed it. Afterwards, the Year 12 Dean who was hosting the event talked us through the meaning and explained that it was a piece by a Haitian composer about three drums who were arguing as to which made the best music but eventually agreed that the best music came from when they performed together.

And that's how I felt about the first forty years of my life – I enjoyed it, I didn't fully understand or appreciate it, and I really would've benefitted from having it explained to me.

Bronnie Ware, a Palliative Health Carer, wrote a book based on her observations of the regrets expressed by the dying.

The top 5 were:

1. I wish I'd had the courage to live a life true to myself and not the life others expected of me,

2. I wish I hadn't worked so hard,

3. I wish I'd had the courage to express my feelings,

4. I wish I had stayed in touch with my friends,

5. I wish that I had let myself be happier

You don't have to give everything up to live longer and better and more productively. You don't have to give anything up. (Except smoking and sunbathing.) Little things can make big differences but you have to do them, not just know them. Keep to a schedule. Move throughout the day. Eat real food. Reduce inflammation. Find or move towards work or a cause that gives you fulfilment, a sense of being valued, being cared for and being liked. Do one thing a day that is likeable. Floss one tooth.

We can't do the easy media headline thing and look at one variable in isolation or look at one fact outside of a context. In 1909, 82% of the fat we consumed in our diets was animal fat. That year, death from heart disease accounted for less than 10% of all deaths. In 2013, 34% of the fat we consume in our diets is animal fat. But now the percentage of deaths attributed to heart disease is greater than 45%. In isolation and without context, we could conclude that eating less animal fat has led to a quadrupling of heart disease deaths. We need to look at other factors such as inactivity and the role of sugar, refined carbohydrates and the other fats on the table. And our mental conditioning that drives behaviours such as over-eating, over-working or avoiding new challenges.

Three quarters of the potential causes of our death and health decline are within our control, within the control of our fingers, feet and forks. Work out specifically and vividly why and for who you'd like to live longer and healthier, Then, make a plan. Do a lot of little things at once. Keep it simple. Get others involved. Start tiny habits linked to your pre-existing habits.

When you _____, you will _____.

You probably knew all this before you read this book. But **do it**. Don't just know it.

Control   *3 Month Goal*

Today's Tiny Habit

- Move

- Eat

- Sleep

- Think

- Learn

- Challenge

- Connect

- Believe

- Hang

- Chill

- Care
Touch

Of all the choices of things to do and tools to try in this book, the choices are yours. Even doing nothing and staying with the same lifestyle and potential health span you have now is a valid choice. But you can't whine about the consequences though. That's the deal.

As a result of the research I've discovered and the people I've interviewed, here are some of my new choices:

- Reorganising my workspace to force far more standing and moving as part of my daily routine,

- Minimise my sugar intake,

- Routine-ise my sleep schedule,

- Disempower my inner critic by giving him the voice of a drunken dickhead,

- Get back into a few hours of guitar a week as a learning challenge to stimulate my brain's plasticity,

- Interview a new person a month for my writing but also to extend my connections,

- Create a rigidly adhered-to weekly family dining event,

- Create and maintain a garden at my new house that requires physical effort,

- Extend the range of causes for whom I help raise funds via 'The Grin Reaper' comedy show.

At the end of my comedy festival show that started the process that led to this book, my conclusion was that the best thing you could do to add ten quality years to your life, and the lives of those you love, was to have a drink and prepare a meal with friends and family every day after a hard but productive workday, then enjoy that meal with those same people having a laugh, reflecting on the day and the past, and talking about plans for the future.

It's never too late to start. It's always too soon to stop.

There's a ton of advice in this book, none better than that. Don't just know it, *do it*. Try. See what happens. If it works, tell your friends. If it doesn't, keep it to yourself. (No one likes a whinger.)

Thank you. Goodnight.

About Terry Williams

Terry Williams is a speaker, trainer and facilitator based in Auckland, New Zealand. He also has a sideline as a stand-up comedian.

His first book was about life skills for young people told in an accessible and non-preachy style. His second, for workplace leaders, was about workplace engagement and motivation. He speaks and trains on a range of topics but, broadly, they all relate to people engagement. If he makes any claims to being an expert on anything at all, it is people engagement.

Recently moved to a rural lifestyle block, his writing time is being impacted by horses and chickens, although he is pretty sure there is a workplace productivity metaphor somewhere amongst the chickens.

www.terrywilliams.info

Bibliography

100 Foods to Stay Young: *Charlotte Watts*

100+: How the Coming Age Of Longevity Will Change Everything: *Sonia Arrison*

121 Ways to Live 121 Years   *Ronald Klatz*

20 Years Younger: *Bob Greene*

59 Seconds *Richard Wiseman*

7 Secrets to Beauty, Health & Longevity: *Nicholas Perricone*

A Long Bright Future: *Laura L Carstensen*

A Ton Of Spirit: Australian Centenarians Talk: *Penny Smith*

Ageless Body Timeless Mind   *Deepak Chopra*

Age-Proof Your Body: *Elizabeth Somers*

Amortality: The Pleasures & Perils of Living Agelessly: *Catherine Mayer*

Ancient Secret Of The Fountain Of Youth Book 2: *Pete Kelder*

Anti-Aging Handbook:Practical Steps To Staying Youthful: *Geraldine Mitton*

Antifragile: Things That Gain From Disorder: *Nassim Taleb*

Bombshell: Explosive Medical Secrets That Will Redefine Aging: *Suzanne Somers*

Buck Up: The Real Bloke's Guide to Getting Healthy And Living Longer: *Grant Schofield*

Can We Live 150 Years? *MikhailTombak*

Celebrate 100: *Steve Franklin*

Chasing Life: *Sanjay Gupta*

Cheat The Clock: How New Science Can Help You Look And Feel Younger : *Margaret Webb Pressler*

Counter Clockwise: Mindful Health & The Power Of Possibility: *Ellen JLanger*

Disease-Proof: The Remarkable Truth About What Makes Us Well: *David L Katz*

Don't Just Do Something, Sit There: *Wallace Chapman*

Eat Move Sleep: *Tom Rath*

Ending Aging : *Aubrey de Grey*

Eternity Soup: Inside the Quest To End Aging: *Greg Critser*

Fantastic Voyage: Live Long Enough to Live Forever: *Ray Kurzwell*

Fat Land: How Americans Became the Fattest People In The World: *Greg Critser*

Forever Young: A Cultural History of Longevity: *Lucian Boia*

Happy Money: The Science of Smarter Spending: *Elizabeth Dunn*

Health, Wellbeing & Environment in Aoteroa New Zealand: *Susan Shaw*

Help Yourself to Living Longer: *Paul Jenner*

How to Live Forever or Die Trying: *Bryan Appleyard*

Hundreds of Ways to Live To Be 100: *Maoshing Ni*

I Is For Influence: *Robert N Yeung*

In Defence Of Food: *Michael Pollan*

Influence: The Psychology of Persuasion: *Robert B Caialdini*

Integrative Wellness Rules: *Jim Nicolai*

Kick Up Your Heels Before You're Too Short To Wear Them: *Loretta LaRoche*

The Book of Immortality: *Adam Leith Gollner*

The Elephant and The Flea: *Charles Handy*

The End of Illness: *David B Agus*

The Essence of Health: The Seven Pillars Of Wellbeing: *Craig Hassed*

The How of Happiness: *Sonja Lyubomirsky*

The Immortality Edge: *Michael Fossel*

The Long Life Equation: *Trisha Macnair*

The Long Tomorrow: *Michael R Rose*

The Longevity Bible: *Gary Small*

The Longevity Factor: *Joseph Maroon*

The Longevity Prescription: *Robert N Butler*

The Longevity Project: *Howard Friedman*

The Longevity Revolution: The Benefits and Challenges of Living A Long Time: *Robert N Butler*

The Old Man's Guide to Health and Longer Life: *John Hill*

The Primal Blueprint: *Mark Sisson*

The Roadmap To 100v*Walter M Bortz II*

The Second Brain: Your Gut Has A Mind of Its Own: *Michael Gershon*

The Wellness Revolution: *Paul Zane Pilzer*

The Youth Pill: Scientists at The Brink of An Anti-Aging Revolution: *David Stipp*

Think Before You Swallow: N*oel O'Hare*

Thrive: Finding Happiness the Blue Zones Way: *Dan Buettner*

Train Your Brain to Get Thin: *Melinda Boyd*

Ultimate Wellness: The 3-Step Plan: *Kerryn Phelps*

Live, Work, Love

Well Being: The Five Essential Elements: *Tom Rath*

Why Do People Get Ill? : *Darian Leader*

Why Men Die First: *Marriane J Legato*

You Are What You Eat: *Carina Norris*

You: Staying Young: *Michael F Roizen*

You: The Owner's Manual: *Michael F Roizen*

Younger Next Year: *Henry S Lodge*

Younger You: *Eric R Braverman*

www.ingramcontent.com/pod-product-compliance
Lightning Source LLC
Chambersburg PA
CBHW062119280526
45788CB00012B/245